Geriatric Dentistry

Editors

LISA A. THOMPSON
LEONARD J. BRENNAN

DENTAL CLINICS OF NORTH AMERICA

www.dental.theclinics.com

October 2014 • Volume 58 • Number 4

ELSEVIER

1600 John F. Kennedy Boulevard • Suite 1800 • Philadelphia, Pennsylvania, 19103-2899

http://www.dental.theclinics.com

DENTAL CLINICS OF NORTH AMERICA Volume 58, Number 4
October 2014 ISSN 0011-8532, ISBN: 978-0-323-32605-6

Editor: John Vassallo; j.vassallo@elsevier.com
Developmental Editor: Yonah Korngold

Dental Clinics of North America (ISSN 0011-8532) is published quarterly by Elsevier Inc., 360 Park Avenue South, New York, NY 10010-1710. Months of issue are January, April, July, and October. Business and Editorial Offices: 1600 John F. Kennedy Boulevard, Suite 1800, Philadelphia, PA 19103-2899. Periodicals postage paid at New York, NY and additional mailing offices. Subscription prices are $280.00 per year (domestic individuals), $485.00 per year (domestic institutions), $135.00 per year (domestic students/residents), $340.00 per year (Canadian individuals), $628.00 per year (Canadian institutions), $410.00 per year (international individuals), $628.00 per year (international institutions), and $200.00 per year (international and Canadian students/residents). International air speed delivery is included in all Clinics subscription prices. All prices are subject to change without notice. **POSTMASTER:** Send address changes to Dental Clinics of North America, Elsevier Health Sciences Division, Subscription Customer Service, 3251 Riverport Lane, Maryland Heights, MO 63043. **Customer Service (orders, claims, online, change of address): Elsevier Health Sciences Division, Subscription Customer Service, 3251 Riverport Lane, Maryland Heights, MO 63043. Tel: 1-800-654-2452 (U.S. and Canada). Fax: 314-447-8029. E-mail: journalscustomer service-usa@elsevier.com (for print support); journalsonlinesupport-usa@elsevier.com (for online support).**

Reprints. For copies of 100 or more, of articles in this publication, please contact the Commercial Reprints Department, Elsevier Inc., 360 Park Avenue South, New York, NY 10010-1710. Tel.: 212-633-3874; Fax: 212-633-3820; E-mail: reprints@elsevier.com.

The Dental Clinics of North America is covered in MEDLINE/PubMed (Index Medicus), Current Contents/Clinical Medicine, ISI/BIOMED and Clinahl.

Printed in the United States of America.

Contributors

EDITORS

LISA A. THOMPSON, DMD
Program Director, Fellowship in Geriatric Dentistry, Department of Oral Health Policy and Epidemiology, Harvard School of Dental Medicine, Boston, Massachusetts

LEONARD J. BRENNAN, DMD
Co-director, Fellowship in Geriatric Dentistry, Department of Oral Health Policy and Epidemiology, Harvard School of Dental Medicine, Boston, Massachusetts

AUTHORS

ALAN P. ABRAMS, MD, MPH
Assistant Professor of Medicine, Harvard Medical School; Program Director, Geriatric Medical Fellowship Program, Division of Gerontology, Beth Israel Deaconess Medical Center, Boston, Massachusetts

NONA AGHAZADEH-SANAI, DDS
Geriatric Dentistry Fellow, Department of Oral Health Policy and Epidemiology, Harvard School of Dental Medicine, Boston, Massachusetts

GREGORY K. AN, DDS, MPH
Dentist, Private Practice, Redwood City, California

LYNN ANN BETHEL, RDH, MPH
Consultant and Former Dental Director, Commonwealth of Massachusetts, Reno, Nevada

LEONARD J. BRENNAN, DMD
Co-director, Fellowship in Geriatric Dentistry, Department of Oral Health Policy and Epidemiology, Harvard School of Dental Medicine, Boston, Massachusetts

MARIA C. DOLCE, PhD, RN, CNE
Associate Professor, School of Nursing, Bouvé College of Health Sciences, Northeastern University, Boston, Massachusetts

CHESTER W. DOUGLASS, DMD, PhD
Professor, Department of Epidemiology, Harvard School of Public Health; Professor Emeritus, Department of Oral Health Policy and Epidemiology, Harvard School of Dental Medicine, Boston, Massachusetts

PAULA K. FRIEDMAN, DDS, MSD, MPH
Professor; Director, Geriatrics and Gerontology, Department of General Dentistry, Boston University Goldman School of Dental Medicine, Boston, Massachusetts

TERRY T. FULMER, PhD, RN, FAAN
Professor, School of Nursing, Professor and Dean, Bouvé College of Health Sciences, Northeastern University; Professor, Public Policy and Urban Affairs, College of Social Sciences and Humanities, Northeastern University, Boston, Massachusetts

MONIK C. JIMÉNEZ, SM, ScD
Associate Epidemiologist, Division of Preventive Medicine, Department of Medicine, Brigham and Women's Hospital; Instructor, Harvard Medical School, Boston, Massachusetts

STEVEN L. KARPAS, DMD
Clinical Assistant Professor, Department of General Dentistry, Boston University Goldman School of Dental Medicine, Boston, Massachusetts

LAURA B. KAUFMAN, DMD
Clinical Assistant Professor, Department of General Dentistry, Boston University Goldman School of Dental Medicine; Section of Geriatrics, Boston Medical Center, Boston, Massachusetts

ESTHER E. KIM, DMD, MPH
Program Coordinator and Dental Public Health Resident, New York State Department of Health, Bureau of Dental Health, Albany, New York

KARI A. LINDEFJELD CALABI, DMD
Geriatric Dentistry Fellow, Department of Oral Health Policy and Epidemiology, Harvard School of Dental Medicine, Boston, Massachusetts

SHAN MOHAMMED, MD, MPH, FAAFP
Clinical Associate Professor, Department of Health Sciences, Bouvé College of Health Sciences, Northeastern University, Boston, Massachusetts

ELLA M. OONG, DMD, MPH
Dentist, Private Practice, Redwood City, California

ATHENA PAPAS, DMD, PhD
Johansen Professor of Dental Research; Head, Division of Oral Medicine, Department of Oral Pathology, Oral Medicine and Craniofacial Pain, Tufts University School of Dental Medicine, Boston, Massachusetts

LAURA SAN MARTIN, DDS, PhD, MDPH
Department of Stomatology, School of Dentistry, University of Seville, Seville, Spain

FRANK A. SCANNAPIECO, DMD, PhD
Professor and Chair, Department of Oral Biology, School of Dental Medicine, University at Buffalo - The State University of New York, Buffalo, New York

CHARLES M. SEITZ, DDS, MPH
Clinical Instructor, Harvard School of Dental Medicine, Boston, Massachusetts; Private Practice, Watertown, Massachusetts

KENNETH SHAY, DDS, MS
Director, Geriatrics and Extended Care Services, US Department of Veterans Affairs, Ann Arbor, Michigan

MABI L. SINGH, DMD, MS
Associate Professor and Director, Dry Mouth Clinic; Department of Oral Pathology, Oral Medicine, Craniofacial Pain Center, Tufts University School of Dental Medicine, Boston, Massachusetts

JASON STRAUSS, MD
Geriatric Psychiatry, CHA Whidden Hospital Campus, Cambridge Health Alliance, Everett, Massachusetts

BRIAN J. SWANN, DDS, MPH
Clinical Instructor, Department of Oral Health Policy and Epidemiology, Harvard School of Dental Medicine, Boston, Massachusetts; Oral Health Department, Cambridge Health Alliance Windsor Street Health Center, Cambridge, Massachusetts

MARY TAVARES, DMD, MPH
Program Director, Dental Public Health, Department of Oral Health Policy and Epidemiology, Harvard School of Dental Medicine, Boston, Massachusetts; Senior Clinical Investigator, Department of Applied Oral Sciences, The Forsyth Institute, Cambridge, Massachusetts

LISA A. THOMPSON, DMD
Program Director, Fellowship in Geriatric Dentistry, Department of Oral Health Policy and Epidemiology, Harvard School of Dental Medicine, Boston, Massachusetts

Contents

socioeconomic level, and sex. Lack of training in treating medically complex patients, economic factors including absence of coverage for oral health services in Medicare and as a required service for adults in Medicaid, and attitudinal issues on the part of patients, caregivers, and providers contribute to barriers to care for older adults. In addition to the impact of oral health on overall health, oral health impacts quality of life and social and employment opportunities.

Poor oral hygiene has been suggested to be a risk factor for aspiration pneumonia in the institutionalized and disabled elderly. Control of oral biofilm formation in these populations reduces the numbers of potential respiratory pathogens in the oral secretions, which in turn reduces the risk for pneumonia. Together with other preventive measures, improved oral hygiene helps to control lower respiratory infections in frail elderly hospital and nursing home patients.

One of the major side effects of medications prescribed to elderly patients is the qualitative and quantitative alteration of saliva (salivary hypofunction). Saliva plays a pivotal role in the homeostasis of the oral cavity because of its protective and functional properties, including facilitating speech, swallowing, enhancing taste, buffering and neutralizing intrinsic and extrinsic acid, remineralizing teeth, maintaining the oral mucosal health, preventing overgrowth of noxious microorganisms, and xerostomia. With salivary hypofunction, a plethora of complications arise, resulting in decreased quality of life. The anticholinergic effects of medications can be overcome, and the oral cavity can be restored to normalcy.

The US population is at the beginning of a significant demographic shift; the American geriatric population is burgeoning, and average longevity is projected to increase in the coming years. Elder adults are affected by numerous chronic conditions, such as diabetes, hypertension, osteoarthritis, osteoporosis, cardiovascular diseases, and cerebrovascular diseases. These older adults need special dental care and an improved understanding of the complex interactions of oral disease and systemic chronic diseases that can complicate their treatment. Oral diseases have strong associations with systemic diseases, and poor oral health can worsen the impact of systemic diseases.

Worldwide incidences of degenerative cognitive diseases are increasing as the population ages. This decline in mental function frequently causes behavioral changes that directly affect oral health. The loss of interest and ability to complete the simple tasks of brushing and flossing can cause a rapid development of hard and soft tissue diseases that result in decreased function and increased dental pain. The challenge for the dental community is to understand and to identify the early signs of cognitive dysfunction so as to develop a rational treatment strategy that allows patients to comfortably maintain their teeth for as long as possible.

Oral health inequities for older adults warrant new models of interprofessional education and collaborative practice. The Innovations in Interprofessional Oral Health: Technology, Instruction, Practice and Service curricular model at Bouvé College of Health Sciences aims to transform health professions education and primary care practice to meet global and local oral health challenges. Innovations in simulation and experiential learning help to advance interprofessional education and integrate oral health care as an essential component of comprehensive primary health care. The Program of All-Inclusive Care for the Elderly clinic is an exemplary model of patient-centeredness and interprofessional collaborative practice for addressing unmet oral health needs of its patient population.

Access to and reducing disparities in oral health for older adults is a complex problem that requires innovative strategies. In addition to offering dental services in alternative settings, such as senior centers, places that are familiar to older adults, and where physical limitations can be better accommodated, alternatives to the traditional provider should be considered. Many states are changing laws and practice acts to allow dental hygienists to provide preventive services without the supervision of a dentist. Also, collaborations between dental and non-dental professionals can be a successful strategy for increasing access to oral health care for this high-risk population.

DENTAL CLINICS OF NORTH AMERICA

DOWNLOAD
Free App!

Review Articles
THE CLINICS

NOW AVAILABLE FOR YOUR iPhone and iPad

Preface

Geriatric Dentistry

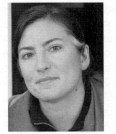 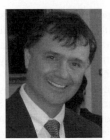

Lisa A. Thompson, DMD   Leonard J. Brennan, DMD
Editors

Good oral health is increasingly recognized today as an integral part of the total health care picture that helps ensure well-being. Health care providers are beginning to understand that poor oral health affects the course of many systemic diseases and additionally has a strong association in the development of other diseases. Consequently, poor oral health is considered a risk factor for poor overall health.

As advances in medicine have extended the life span of our older population, it is very important for us to remember the words of President John F. Kennedy, "it is not enough for a great nation to have added new years to life. Our objective must be to add new life to those years." Seniors can expect to live longer today than ever before. The burden of oral diseases tends to increase with age. With the evolution and developments within the science and understanding of geriatric dentistry, early prevention and treatment will reduce oral disease and aid in the management of systemic diseases. The former Surgeon General David Satcher emphasized the very important need to reconnect the mouth to the rest our body and to see it as an integral part of total health.

Senior oral health care must be interdisciplinary and interprofessional to provide the most efficient and effective results. Everyone involved in the overall treatment for the elderly has an important piece of the health care puzzle to manage through education, communication, and assessment. As patients age, dentists are continuously challenged to alter their treatment plans to provide rational care to accommodate physical and mental health deterioration.

This issue, "Geriatric Dentistry," recognizes the challenges that our aging population face and offers new evidence-based insights on senior oral health care. Dr Chester W. Douglass and Monik C. Jiménez begin their article by updating us on the aging geriatric population, demographics, oral health care utilization, and recommendations to connect oral health care to primary care. Today's older adults are tremendously varied in health status; Drs Alan P. Abrams and Lisa A. Thompson walk us through

Dent Clin N Am 58 (2014) xi–xiii
http://dx.doi.org/10.1016/j.cden.2014.07.007
0011-8532/14/$ – see front matter © 2014 Elsevier Inc. All rights reserved.

normal physiologic changes in systemic and oral health that occur with aging to remind us of the challenges aging alone presents, in the absence of disease. Drs Ella Oong and Gregory An highlight the importance of comprehensive diagnosis and treatment planning and demonstrate how it differs from treatment planning in younger cohorts.

As the geriatric population ages, becomes more diverse, lives longer, retains their teeth longer, and presents with multiple chronic health conditions, we face an increase in oral health disparities. Drs Paula K. Friedman, Laura B. Kaufman, and Steven Karpas provide data on disparities in dental decay and tooth loss, the consequence of these disparities, and the challenges facing the dental workforce to treat this population. As oral health research continues to provide links between oral and systemic health, Drs Frank A. Scannapieco and Kenneth Shay explain the pathogenesis and risk factors of aspiration pneumonia and its prevalence in older adults and provide interventions to reduce the risk in this vulnerable population. With the geriatric population among the highest users of prescription medications, Drs Athena Papas and Mabi Singh consider the clinical implications of polypharmacy and provide us with insight into how salivary function affects oral health of older adults. In the article, "Oral and Systemic Health," Drs Mary Tavares, Kari Lindefjeld, and Laura San Martin pull together many of the concepts that have been discussed in previous articles and provide clinical oral health recommendations for several of the most common systemic diseases. Drs Leonard Brennan and Jason Strauss cover the topic of cognitive impairment relative to oral health and stress the importance of early intervention and education by caregivers in the care of the oral and overall health of older adults.

We close this issue with two exciting articles that provide strategies and innovation in education and health care delivery to address the disparities in oral health care for older adults. First, Drs Maria C. Dolce, Nona Aghazadeh-Sanai, Shan Mohammed, and Terry T. Fulmer write about interprofessional curricula and programs that are effective in introducing oral health to primary care and allied health care and the importance of these programs in addressing health disparities. Finally, Lynn A. Bethel and Drs Esther E. Kim, Charlie M. Seitz, and Brian J. Swann cover trends in dental education and practice and highlight several innovative approaches that address issues of access to care and bridging the gap between dental and medical education and practice.

In summary, it is our hope that this issue will improve the knowledge of health care providers that participate in senior health and help promote the importance of a team-based approach to early treatment and management of disease through rational planning. Our goal has been to update readers and clinicians on topics in geriatric dentistry, provide recommendations for caring for older adults, and highlight shifts in oral health care delivery through innovation and collaboration. Ultimately, an integrated approach to care in geriatric dentistry improves the dignity and quality of life for our aging population.

We want to thank all the authors for collaborating on this issue and bringing relevant and evidence-based information to the field of geriatric dentistry.

Lisa A. Thompson, DMD
Geriatric Dentistry
Department of Oral Health Policy and Epidemiology
Harvard School of Dental Medicine
188 Longwood Avenue
Boston, MA 02115, USA

Leonard J. Brennan, DMD
Geriatric Dentistry
Department of Oral Health Policy and Epidemiology
Harvard School of Dental Medicine
188 Longwood Avenue
Boston, MA 02115, USA

E-mail addresses:
Lisa_Thompson@hsdm.harvard.edu (L.A. Thompson)
Leonard_Brennan@hsdm.harvard.edu (L.J. Brennan)

Erratum

 CrossMark

In the January 2014 issue (Volume 58, number 1), in the article "Caries Management by Risk Assessment Care Paths for Prosthodontic Patients: Oral Microbial Control and Management," by Hamilton H. Le and Roy T. Yanase, the authors inadvertently failed to attribute information on pages 231 and 234 to reference 19. The authors apologize for this oversight and have provided new text to properly recognize the original source.

The new text should read:

Previous studies highlight a reduction in acid production in bacterial cells, by way of the inhibition of a key enzyme, enolase. Enolase, a glycolytic enzyme, has a crucial role in the conversion of 2-P-glycerate (2-PG) to P-enolpyruvate (PEP). Hamilton found a decrease in the production of PEP in the presence of the fluoride anion.[19]

Hamilton goes on to show that the accumulation of F^- in the bacterial cell cytoplasm is dependent on the transport of hydrogen fluoride (HF) through a transmembrane pH difference, or pH gradient, characteristic only in metabolically active cells. Once inside the cell, the basic environment of the cytoplasm leads to the dissociation of HF back to H^+ cations and F^- anions, thereby acidifying the cytoplasm of the cell and reducing the pH gradient. Current studies have revealed that, in addition to enolase, F^- also has an inhibitory effect on the membrane bound proton pump adenosine triphosphatase (ATPase). Inhibition of the pump results in the inability of a cell to reestablish a pH gradient, reducing the cell's ability to transport solutes through mechanisms that are dependent on this gradient. Despite the dual versatility of fluoride to dissociate proton gradients as well as prevent their regeneration there remains a lack of consensus about the antimicrobial effects of F^- and its contributions to caries management.[19]

REFERENCE

19. Hamilton IR. Biochemical effects of fluoride on oral bacteria. J Dent Res 1990;(69 Spec No):660–7.

Dent Clin N Am 58 (2014) xv
http://dx.doi.org/10.1016/j.cden.2014.07.006
0011-8532/14/$ – see front matter © 2014 Elsevier Inc. All rights reserved.

dental.theclinics.com

Our Current Geriatric Population

Demographic and Oral Health Care Utilization

Chester W. Douglass, DMD, PhD[a,b,*], Monik C. Jiménez, SM, ScD[c]

KEYWORDS

- Old age • Geriatric • Living arrangement • Population trends
- Dental care and demand • Primary care

KEY POINTS

- Changes in the US population age distribution owing to the baby boom generation will result in a substantial increase in the geriatric population over the next 30 years.
- Aging can be defined in chronologic, physical, and social terms, reflecting changes in an individual's participation within their sociocultural context or physical or functional capabilities.
- Older adults are retaining greater numbers of their natural dentition, which will result in a greater unmet need and effective demand for dental care.
- Dentists should be more closely linked to primary care or provide primary care in the dental office.

DEFINING OLD AGE

There is no one accepted definition or threshold for old age, and yet there are a multitude of terms describing this life stage and progressions within it. Terms such as *old*, *elderly*, and *senior*, are often used to refer social constructs of chronologic age that mark changes in an individual's participation within their sociocultural context or physical or functional capabilities (**Box 1**). Other terms such as *successful aging*, *frail elderly*, and *oldest old* refer to loosely defined phases of the older age life stage with unique considerations.

The authors have nothing to disclose.
[a] Department of Epidemiology, Harvard School of Public Health, 677 Huntington Avenue, Boston, MA 02115, USA; [b] Department of Oral Health Policy and Epidemiology, Harvard School of Dental Medicine, 188 Longwood Avenue, Boston, MA 02115, USA; [c] Division of Preventive Medicine, Department of Medicine, Brigham and Women's Hospital, Harvard Medical School, 900 Commonwealth Avenue, 3rd Floor, Boston, MA 02215, USA
* Corresponding author. Department of Oral Health Policy and Epidemiology, Harvard School of Dental Medicine, 188 Longwood Avenue, Boston, MA 02115.
E-mail address: chester_douglass@hsdm.harvard.edu

Dent Clin N Am 58 (2014) 717–728
http://dx.doi.org/10.1016/j.cden.2014.06.001
0011-8532/14/$ – see front matter © 2014 Elsevier Inc. All rights reserved.

> **Box 1**
> **Glossary of terms**
>
> Old age: Associated terms used to refer to social constructs of chronologic age, which mark changes in an individual's participation within their sociocultural context or physical or functional capabilities.
>
> Frail elderly: Older individuals with functional or physical impairments influencing activities of daily living.
>
> Vulnerable older adults: Older adults at risk of frailty, morbidity, or mortality within 2 years, potentially identified by risk factors such as age, self-reported health status, and physical and functional status.
>
> Oldest old: The upper age categories within a population. The age thresholds that identify this group depend on the particular population and range from 75 to 90 years.
>
> Successful aging: The least decline in physical or mental function with chronologic age.

Although the biology of aging is immutable, the threshold at which we decide an individual has reached old age varies substantially across countries and cultures. In most developed countries, 60 to 65 years, the age of retirement or pension benefits, has become synonymous with the onset of old age or senior status. In developing countries, the transition to older age may be the attainment of social roles assigned to older individuals or the loss of roles because of loss of physical of functional limitations.[1] The United Nations agreed that the threshold for older age is ≥60 years; however, variation in disease, socioeconomic conditions, and access to basic needs may substantially influence the equivalency of age groups across various populations.[2]

The term *frail elderly* is often used to refer to older individuals with functional or physical impairments; however, the criteria used to define frail vary depending on the utilization of the definition, whether for research or resource allocation. For example, when used for research purposes, frailty has been defined broadly in terms of physical impairments such as muscle weakness, slow walking speed, exhaustion, low physical activity, and little tolerance of physical stress.[3] However, for the purposes of resource allocation for community-based care services, Congress defines frail elderly based on activity of daily living impairments. Similarly for housing allocation, the US Department of Housing and Urban Development defines such individuals as those who are unable to perform "at least three activities of daily living comprising of eating, bathing, grooming, dressing, or home management activities."[4] Other terms such as *vulnerable older adults* have been used to identify those who may be at risk of frailty, morbidity, or mortality within 2 years.[5] A score based on older age, self-reported health status, and physical and functional limitations has been used to identify vulnerable older adults and assess appropriate delivery of care.[5]

The term *oldest old* refers to those older individuals above a particular age cutoff defined at 75,[6] 80,[7,8] 85,[9] and even 90 years.[10] In the United States, those 85 to 94 years were the most rapidly growing elderly age group, increasing from 3.9 to 5.1 million in 2010 and expected to exceed 19 million by 2050.[11] The appropriate threshold for oldest old depends on the age distribution of the underlying population, with the US Census using ≥85 years as the threshold for oldest old.[11] Much research among oldest old populations centers on factors of successful aging. The term *successful aging* generally refers to the least decline in physical or mental function with chronologic aging. Rowe and Kahn[12] highlight the intersection of lifestyle choices, engagement in life, and remaining disease-free years in successful aging and underscore the influence of self-efficacy. Hence, as the US and global population continue to age, substantial research should focus on what behavioral, dietary, lifestyle and psychosocial factors may foster a longer, healthier, and active life.

LIVING ARRANGEMENTS

The living arrangements of older adults often change because of retirement, illness, or functional limitations. Although many individuals remain living in their own homes with or without home health care, others may opt for retirement villages or assisted living communities. Nursing homes may be chosen in the event of debilitating illness and hospice for end-of-life care.

Research from the Health and Retirement Study (HRS), a nationally representative study of older Americans, reported that nearly 79% of participants continued to live in a home they or their spouse owned. Although the prevalence of home ownership declined with age, home ownership remained at nearly 50% among those ≥85 years.[13] According to US Census data, approximately 54% of adults ≥65 years live with their spouse, 30% live alone, 13% live with relative, and 2.3% with nonrelatives.[14] Importantly, among those ≥65 years, women were substantially more likely to be widowed than men (44.3% vs 14.3%, respectively).[14]

Living with children is an important alternative for many older adults. Estimates from the HRS reported 11% of participants living with a child, however, and additional 51% reported at least 1 child living within 10 miles. However, African-American, Latino, and Asian older adults were more likely than non-Hispanic whites to live with relatives according to US Census data.[14] Other research suggests a higher percentage of baby boomers anticipate living with adult children than those from previous decades.[15]

Home health care provides a wide range of medical and nonmedical services in the home setting, allowing individuals to remain in their home while maintaining autonomy and independence.[16] Services offered include skilled nursing services, assistance with activities of daily living, physical therapy, homemaking, wound care, and dietary counseling.[16] Research from the National Home and Hospice Care Survey reported 1.46 million US home health care patients in 2007.[16] Patients were more likely to be ≥65 years (69%), female (64%), and white (82%). Furthermore, male home health care patients were nearly 3 times as likely as female home health care patients to have a spouse as their primary care provider, whereas women were about twice as likely as men to have a child or nonspouse as a primary care provider.[16]

Assisted living facilities (ALFs) are an important community-based long-term care alternative for adults requiring assistance with a wide range of activities from those of daily living to chronic disease and physical impairment.[17] However, there is no formal definition characterizing assisted living services. Furthermore, because they are not subsidized by public funds, these facilities are not tightly regulated by state-wide licensing; hence, substantial variations exist across facilities.[18] Moreover, no data are available on operating ALFs at the national level. Research suggests that approximately 38,000 facilities serving up to 975,000 units (units may contain multiple beds [eg, married individuals]) were operational as of 2007; this is more than double the number of nursing home facilities but with substantially lower capacity.[17] As expected, ALFs track tightly with private resources (income, educational attainment, and area wealth), as this care option is primarily supported by personal financing.

Nursing homes provide the next level of care by administering care for chronically ill or disabled individuals in a residential environment.[19] The probability of residing in a nursing home increases with age, and approximately 1.5 million adults, or 4% of those age ≥65 years, currently reside in US nursing homes.[14,20] Among HRS participants, the percentage of those 75 to 84 years living in nursing homes or ALFs was 7% and increased to 20% for those ≥85 years in 2002.[13] Nursing homes are required to provide regular assessment reporting on facility performance and complaint investigations. Potential consumers can inquire about nursing facilities through databases maintained by the Centers for Medicare & Medicaid Services.[21]

Hospice care can be a critically important care option for older individuals. Hospice aims to alleviate pain and suffering providing compassionate, emotional, and spiritual support to the terminally ill and their families.[22] In 2011, 1.65 million patients were estimated to receive care under hospice (not all died; some carried over to the following year, and approximately 300,000 were discharged), which comprises approximately 45% of all US deaths.[22] Provision of hospice care can occur in the home, in hospice facilities, and increasingly in nursing homes.[22] Research suggests that hospice patients in nursing homes were primarily female (67%), white (90%), and age ≥85 years (55%).[23]

DEMOGRAPHIC TRENDS

The demography of the older adult population will change dramatically over the next 40 years. This shift is caused largely by the aging of the baby boom generation born between 1946 and 1964 (**Fig. 1**). In 2011 the first cohort of baby boomers turned 65. Now 10,000 baby boomers become 65 every day.[24] This trend will continue unabated for the next 16 years. This age cohort can be seen coming through the society from 1980 (**Fig. 2**) through 2000 (**Fig. 3**) and 2020 (**Fig. 4**) to 2040 (**Fig. 5**). From 2010 to 2050 the elderly population more than doubles from 40.2 million to 86.7 million (**Fig. 6**).[14] As seen in the figures, the baby boomers have reshaped the US population from 1960 to 2020, and their ability to maintain active engaged lifestyles may redefine successful aging over the next 30 years.

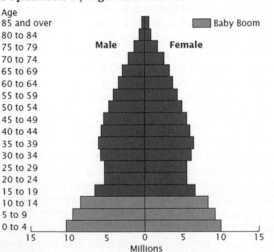

Note: The reference population for these data is the resident population.

Fig. 1. US population by age and sex in 1960. (*From* He W, Sengupta M, Velkoff VA, et al. U.S. Census Bureau, current population reports, P23-209, 65+ in the United States: 2005. Washington, DC: U.S. Government Printing Office; 2005; and *Data from* U.S. Bureau of the Census. 1964, Table 156.)

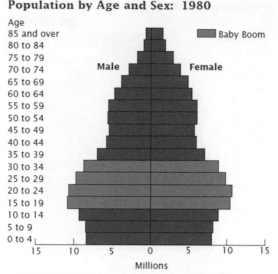

Fig. 2. US population by age and sex in 1980. (*From* He W, Sengupta M, Velkoff VA, et al. U.S. Census Bureau, current population reports, P23-209, 65+ in the United States: 2005. Washington, DC: U.S. Government Printing Office; 2005; and *Data from* U.S. Bureau of the Census. 1983, Table 44.)

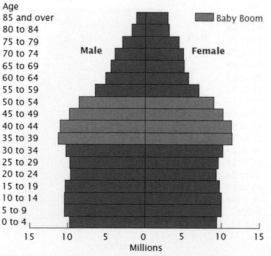

Fig. 3. US population by age and sex in 2000. (*From* He W, Sengupta M, Velkoff VA, et al. U.S. Census Bureau, current population reports, P23-209, 65+ in the United States: 2005. Washington, DC: U.S. Government Printing Office; 2005; and *Data from* U.S. Bureau of the Census. 2001, Table PCT12.)

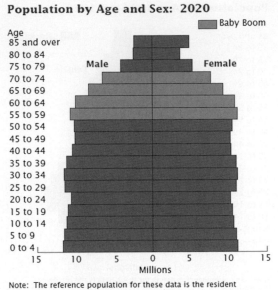

Fig. 4. US population by age and sex in 2020. (*From* He W, Sengupta M, Velkoff VA, et al. U.S. Census Bureau, current population reports, P23-209, 65+ in the United States: 2005. Washington, DC: U.S. Government Printing Office; 2005; and *Data from* U.S. Census Bureau. 2004.)

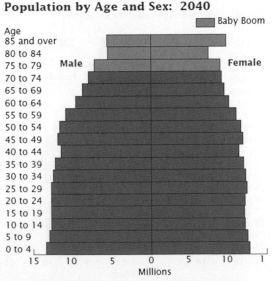

Fig. 5. US population by age and sex in 2040. (*From* He W, Sengupta M, Velkoff VA, et al. U.S. Census Bureau, current population reports, P23-209, 65+ in the United States: 2005. Washington, DC: U.S. Government Printing Office; 2005; and *Data from* U.S. Census Bureau. 2004.)

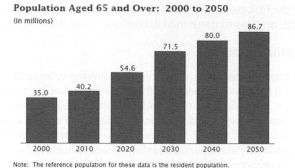

Fig. 6. US population age 65 and older from 2000 to 2050. (*From* He W, Sengupta M, Velkoff VA, et al. U.S. Census Bureau, current population reports, P23-209, 65+ in the United States: 2005. Washington, DC: U.S. Government Printing Office; 2005; *Data from* 2000, U.S. Census Bureau, 2001, Table PCT12; and 2010 to 2050, U.S. Census Bureau, 2004.)

NEED FOR DENTAL CARE

This relentless upward trend of older adults has resulted in projections for dental care needs that have been reported in the literature and summarized here.

Dentures

The percentage of older adults older than 65 years needing a denture is declining because of the retention of natural dentition. However, the number of older adults is increasing so rapidly that the actual number of edentulous arches will increase.[25]

Fixed Prosthodontics

The calculations for partial edentulism are similar. Between 2010 and 2020 the number of hours of provider time needed to treat the removable partial denture and fixed partial denture needs of adults age 65 and older increase dramatically. The retention of more posterior teeth and the emergence of dental implants have created many more cases for which fixed partial dentures are the treatment of choice.[26]

Operative Dentistry

Demographics and epidemiologic trends show that older adult age groups will continue to need operative dentistry services. This age group was born too soon to have benefitted greatly from preventive dentistry.[27]

Endodontics

With increases in fixed prosthodontics come increases in the number of pulp chambers that have been challenged too many times and finally require endodontic therapy. The number of teeth requiring root canal treatment will increase for the older adult cohorts.[28]

Periodontology

With the retention of the natural dentition, older adults will need treatment for chronic periodontal disease. With overall improvements in oral health comes the retention of the natural dentition for the baby boom generation. Ironically, this improvement in number of natural teeth retained will put older adults at greater risk to periodontal disease.[29,30]

The need for dental care will increase for older adults over the next 20 years as the number of adults doubles to more than 80 million.

DENTAL CARE UTILIZATION

Changes in utilization of dental care at retirement among older adults is complex and may be influenced by loss of coverage and lower income leading to less utilization but also an increase in free time potentially leading to increased care seeking. Manski and colleagues,[31] reported that individuals age ≥65 were more likely to seek dental care utilization than those less than 65. However, full retirement "when accompanied by reduced income and dental insurance coverage," was associated with lower utilization of dental services among participants of the HRS.[31] Disparities in dental care utilization by race/ethnicity persist among older adults. African-American and Latino elders exhibited approximately 40% and 60% lower odds of dental visits, respectively, albeit updated data are needed.[32] Research shows that perceived importance of dental care was the primary predictor of dental care utilization, followed by perceived need and number of remaining teeth.[33–35] Furthermore, education status and income play key mediating roles.[36]

Surveys of dental care utilizations are primarily focused on noninstitutionalized individuals and, therefore, do not capture the dental care utilization or needs of nursing home or hospitalized older adults. In a survey among Canadian dentists, only 19% had provided dental care of primarily an emergency nature in nursing homes, despite proximate dental practices. Nearly 25% of the dentists surveyed felt unprepared for treating frail elderly patients with various comorbid conditions.[36] Nursing home and hospitalized patients continue to be a vulnerable population with unique dental health needs.

INTEGRATION WITH PRIMARY CARE

With the number of older adults doubling in the next 25 years, the trends in chronic disease will become a major factor. The following general facts about chronic disease provide a summary of the emerging crisis in chronic disease management.

- 70% of deaths are caused by chronic disease
- 75% of health care expenditures are spent for chronic diseases
- Of those with chronic illness, 25% experience one or more limitations in their daily activities of living.

The most prevalent chronic disease conditions are asthma, diabetes, coronary heart disease, stroke, cancer and, obesity, which is now considered to be a chronic disease. Older adults have the most vulnerability to chronic disease. As a result of disease rates and population trends, the number of people (in millions) with chronic disease will increase (**Table 1**).[37] As the older adult population grows and ages, the prevalence of chronic diseases will increase and become a significant burden for primary care providers.

Primary care consists largely of patient assessment, management of chronic disease, and the maintenance of health by controlling risk factors and improving protective factors for chronic conditions. Traditionally, general practice physicians, family medicine physicians, and pediatricians provide these services. However, medical workforce reports document that fewer medical students are going into primary care practice, choosing rather the procedure based specialties. Given this workforce trend, who will provide primary care? One response is that physician assistants (PA's) and nurse practitioners (NP's) will become the most likely candidates to fill these

Table 1
Current and projected numbers of people with chronic disease (in millions)

Chronic Disease	2010	2050
Asthma, lifetime	40.8	55.8
Asthma, current	25.2	34.4
Diabetes	19.0	26.0
Obesity (body mass index 30+)	111.1	152.0
Coronary heart disease	19.5	26.5
Stroke	8.0	10.9

needs for older adults. However, why shouldn't dentists become the primary care providers for their own patients?

Dentists are well qualified in the basic sciences, and they already need to document the medical history of each patient to provide quality dental care. Dentists could take it one step further to document and then help patients control their risk factors for diabetes, cardiovascular disease, and other chronic conditions. This is the essence of primary care—patient assessment and primary care through risk factor control.

Dentists who provide the core elements of primary care for their older dental patients would be helping to build a stronger, more coordinated and more collaborative health care system for older adults. It would improve the efficiency of the health care

Box 2
Chronic disease risk factors

Self-reported risk factors

1. Age

2. Sex

3. Self-reported race/ethnicity

4. Family history of diabetes

5. Smoking

6. Postmenopausal status

7. Hormone therapy use

Clinically measured risk factors

1. Waist circumference

2. Weight[a]

3. Blood pressure

Biomarkers

1. Hemoglobin A1c

2. Total cholesterol

3. High-density lipoprotein cholesterol

Oral health risk factors

1. Periodontal status

2. Self-reported oral health status

[a] Can be assessed by direct measurement or self-report.

system for geriatric patients. Risk factor control would improve, and ambulatory dental care patients would be better off for it, because their dental and oral health would be integrated with overall medical needs and health concerns.

CLINICAL AND CHRONIC DISEASE RISK FACTORS IDENTIFIABLE IN THE DENTAL PRACTICE

Cardiovascular disease, diabetes, and oral disease share substantial overlap with respect to deleterious clinical and chronic disease risk factors (**Box 2**). Dentists and dental hygienists can play an active role in identifying and aiding in patient risk factor management by assessing easily measured risk factors as part of a routine dental visit. Li and colleagues[38] identified several easily measured risk factors for identifying undiagnosed diabetes in the dental clinic setting: age, self-reported race/ethnicity, waist circumference, family history of diabetes, periodontal status, and self-reported weight and oral health status. Greenberg and colleagues[39] found that a simple cardiovascular disease questionnaire, measured blood pressure, and finger-stick blood testing (ie, lipids, hemoglobin A1c) significantly identified a high prevalence of cardiovascular risk factors according to the Framingham risk score among a dental clinic population otherwise unaware of their cardiovascular disease factor status. This study found not only a high prevalence of risk factors and substantial variation by gender but more importantly the effectiveness of implementation within a routine dental visit. Hence, ample opportunity exists for dental professionals to collaborate in patient systemic risk factor identification and management.

SUMMARY

Driven largely by the baby boom generation born between 1946 and 1964, the shape of the US population has changed dramatically over the last 50 years. Now, this cohort is aging, resulting in a huge increase in the geriatric population over the next 30 years. Aging can be defined in chronologic, physical, and social terms. Frail or vulnerable elders are those who exhibit some kind of medical or mental challenge. These definitions of aging determine the degree to which a person is on the path to successful aging. Half of elders still live at home, but an increasing number live in housing that is coming to be known as the *senior industry* by real estate agents. These retirement villages offer independent living units and retirement villages/assisted living facilities that are commonly linked with a series of nursing home levels and ultimately hospice care. Because of extended longevity and the improvements in oral health, older adults are retaining greater numbers of their natural dentition. Hence, both the unmet need and the effective demand for dental care will increase among the over-65 age groups. Because chronic disease increases with age, the numbers of senior adults living with diabetes, cardiovascular disease, asthma, or other chronic conditions will increase dramatically as the older adult age groups increase to 80 million. With a shortage of primary care physicians, dentists could monitor these chronic diseases in their dental patients and provide assistance in managing their chronic disease risk factors and improving their protective factors. Dental care for older adults should be linked closely with primary health care. Dental care providers can become that link.

REFERENCES

1. Gorman M. Development and the rights of older people. In: Randel JE, editor. The ageing and development report: poverty, independence and the world's older people. London: Earthscan Publications Ltd; 1999. p. 3–21.

2. World Health Organization. Definition of an older or elderly person. Health Statistics and Health Information Systems; 2013.
3. RAND Corporation. Frail elderly; 2011. Available at: http://www.rand.org/health/projects/special-needs-populations-mapping/promising-practices/frail-elderly.html. Accessed December 19, 2013.
4. US Dept of Housing and Urban Development. Glossary of hud terms. Available at: http://www.huduser.org/portal/glossary/glossary_all.html. Accessed December 31, 2013.
5. Shekelle PG, Rubenstein L, Solomon D, et al. Quality of health care received by older adults. Research Briefs. 2004;2013:4. Available at: http://www.rand.org/health/projects/special-needs-populations-mapping/promising-practices/frail-elderly.html.
6. Musso CG, Alvarez Gregori J, Jauregui JR, et al. Creatinine, urea, uric acid, water and electrolytes renal handling in the healthy oldest old. World J Nephrol 2012;1:123–6.
7. Spaniolas K, Trus TL, Adrales GL. Ventral hernia repairs in the oldest-old: high-risk regardless of approach. Surg Endosc 2014;28:1230–7.
8. Liu J, Guo M, Bern-Klug M. Economic stress among adult-child caregivers of the oldest old in china: the importance of contextual factors. J Cross Cult Gerontol 2013;28:465–79.
9. Willems JM, Vlasveld T, den Elzen WP, et al. Performance of cockcroft-gault, mdrd, and ckd-epi in estimating prevalence of renal function and predicting survival in the oldest old. BMC Geriatr 2013;13:113.
10. Mengel-From J, Thinggaard M, Lindahl-Jacobsen R, et al. Clu genetic variants and cognitive decline among elderly and oldest old. PLoS One 2013;8:e79105.
11. Werner CA. The older population: U.S. Department of Commerce, Economics and Statistics Administration; 2011. 2010 Census Briefs.
12. Rowe J, Khan R. Successful aging. New York: Pantheon; 1998.
13. National Institute on Aging. Growing older in America: the health and retirement study. In: National Institutes of Health. Rockville, MD: U.S. Department of Health and Human Services; 2007.
14. He W, Sengupta M, Velkoff VA, DeBarros KA. 65+ in the United States: 2005 current population reports. In: U.S. Census Bureau. Washington, DC: U.S. Government Printing Office; 2005. Current populations reports: special studies. 2005.
15. Robison J, Shugrue N, Fortinsky RH, et al. Long-term supports and services planning for the future: implications from a statewide survey of baby boomers and older adults. Gerontologist 2014;54:297–313.
16. Jones A, Harris-Kojetin L, Valverde R. Characteristics and use of home health care by men and women aged 65 and over. Natl Health Stat Report 2012;(52):1–7.
17. Stevenson DG, Grabowski DC. Sizing up the market for assisted living. Health Aff (Millwood) 2010;29:35–43.
18. Mollica RL. Residential care and assisted living: State oversight practices and state information available to consumers. Agency for Healthcare Research and Quality; 2006.
19. Kim SJ, Park EC, Kim S, et al. The association between quality of care and quality of life in long-stay nursing home residents with preserved cognition. J Am Med Dir Assoc 2014;15:220–5.
20. Centers for Disease Control and Prevention, National Center for Health Statistics. 2004 national nursing home survey, residents, table 13. 2004. Centers for Disease Control and Prevention; 2013. Available at: http://www.cdc.gov/nchs/data/nnhsd/Estimates/nnhs/Estimates_PaymentSource_Tables.pdf. Accessed January 6, 2014.

21. Agency for Healthcare Research and Quality. Section 1: introduction and overview: Residential care and assisted living. Rockville, MD; 2006.
22. National Hospice and Palliative Care Organization. Nhpco facts and figures: Hospice care in America. Alexandria, VA; 2012.
23. Miller SC, Lima J, Gozalo PL, et al. The growth of hospice care in U.S. Nursing homes. J Am Geriatr Soc 2010;58:1481–8.
24. Cohn D, Taylor P. Baby Boomers Approach 65 – Glumly: Survey Findings about America's Largest Generation. Pew research survey reports. Washington, DC: Pew Research Center; 2010.
25. U.S. Census Bureau. U.S. Population projections. National population projections based on census 2000. Available at: http://www.census.gov/population/projections/data/national/natsum.html. Accessed December 15, 2013.
26. Douglass CW, Shih A, Ostry L. Will there be a need for complete dentures in the united states in 2020? J Prosthet Dent 2002;87:5–8.
27. Douglass CW, Watson AJ. Future needs for fixed and removable partial dentures in the united states. J Prosthet Dent 2002;87:9–14.
28. Reinhardt JW, Douglass CW. The need for operative dentistry services: projecting the effects of changing disease patterns. Oper Dent 1989;14:114–20.
29. Douglass CW, Furino A. Balancing dental service requirements and supplies: epidemiologic and demographic evidence. J Am Dent Assoc 1990;121:587–92.
30. Douglass CW. Epidemiology of periodontal disease. Curr Opin Dent 1991;1:12–6.
31. Manski RJ, Moeller J, Schimmel J, et al. Dental care coverage and retirement. J Public Health Dent 2010;70:1–12.
32. Manski RJ, Goodman HS, Reid BC, et al. Dental insurance visits and expenditures among older adults. Am J Public Health 2004;94:759–64.
33. Gilbert GH, Duncan RP, Crandall LA, et al. Older floridians' attitudes toward and use of dental care. J Aging Health 1994;6:89–110.
34. Gilbert GH, Duncan RP, Heft MW, et al. Dental health attitudes among dentate black and white adults. Med Care 1997;35:255–71.
35. Kiyak HA. An explanatory model of older persons' use of dental services. Implications for health policy. Med Care 1987;25:936–52.
36. Kiyak HA, Reichmuth M. Barriers to and enablers of older adults' use of dental services. J Dent Educ 2005;69:975–86.
37. Douglass CW, Shanmugham J. Primary care, the dental profession, and the prevalence of chronic diseases in the united states. Dent Clin North Am 2013;56:699–730.
38. Li S, Williams PL, Douglass CW. Development of a clinical guideline to predict undiagnosed diabetes in dental patients. J Am Dent Assoc 2011;142:28–37.
39. Greenberg BL, Glick M, Goodchild J, et al. Screening for cardiovascular risk factors in a dental setting. J Am Dent Assoc 2007;138:798–804.

Physiology of Aging of Older Adults

Systemic and Oral Health Considerations

Alan P. Abrams, MD, MPH[a,b,*], Lisa A. Thompson, DMD[c]

KEYWORDS

- Physiology • Aging adults • Oral health • Normal aging • Age-dependent changes
- Systemic

KEY POINTS

- Oral health plays a vital role in several functions that contribute to life quality, longevity, and functional independence.
- The oral cavity, when functioning properly, provides and contributes to the enjoyment of taste and smell; the appropriate steps needed for deglutition and nutrition; maintenance of facial anatomy; and self-esteem.
- Older adults differ more from one another physiologically than do younger adults, which makes geriatric care a greater challenge for the clinician.

INTRODUCTION

Much has been written about the nature and extent of the demographic shift taking place in the United States. By 2030 the baby-boomer generation will reconstruct the population pyramid into a population rectangle, with the fastest growing segment of that polygon being the oldest of the old (>85 years). As the population ages it becomes more heterogeneous, with a wider distribution of physiologic reserve for each individual. Cognitive status, chronic multiple diseases, and medications add to the heterogeneity of this physiologically diverse population segment. Normative aging studies demonstrate a wider distribution around the mean in most physiologic measures. In simpler terms, healthy older adults are more unlike each other than equally healthy younger adults in most studies of physiologic function. Though less thoroughly

Conflict of Interest: The authors have nothing to disclose.
[a] Geriatric Medical Fellowship Program, Division of Gerontology, Beth Israel Deaconess Medical Center, 110 Francis Street, Boston, MA 02115, USA; [b] Harvard Medical School, Boston, MA 02115, USA; [c] Fellowship in Geriatric Dentistry, Department of Oral Health Policy and Epidemiology, Harvard School of Dental Medicine, 188 Longwood Avenue, Boston, MA 02115, USA
* Corresponding author. Geriatric Medical Fellowship Program, Division of Gerontology, Beth Israel Deaconess Medical Center, 110 Francis Street, Boston, MA 02115.
E-mail address: aabrams@bidmc.harvard.edu

Dent Clin N Am 58 (2014) 729–738
http://dx.doi.org/10.1016/j.cden.2014.06.002   **dental.theclinics.com**

studied, changes in oral health over the life span seem to observe the same principles of normative physiologic aging that apply to other organ systems and physiologic processes. "Oral aging" is as relevant as any other health care challenge facing an aging society. Many well-studied physiologic functions of the older adult population affect the oral cavity. Many of these physiologic changes contribute to the lower threshold for the development of oral disease, nutritional and swallowing problems, taste and smell impairment, chronic pain, and psychological distress. This article reviews the concepts of physiologic reserve, the normative aging processes of the cardiovascular, neurologic, and musculoskeletal systems that are applicable to oral health, and age-related changes in the oral cavity itself, and reflects on how they may contribute to disease management by oral health care providers. The article is not intended to focus on disease related to aging but rather aims to explore the normal physiologic changes associated with aging dentition and systemic changes related to age, thus enabling clinicians to obtain a better understanding of the presentation of older adults and how it may change their approach to diagnosis and treatment.

PHYSIOLOGY OF AGING

When considering aging physiology, it is first important to understand that we are unsure of where aging ends and disease begins. Wherever that line divides normative physiologic changes of aging and disease, it is clear that aging alone changes the physiologic threshold for any individual to withstand physiologic challenges, whether brought on by medications, stressful interventions such as surgery, severe environmental conditions, or other illness. What we do know is that, in the elderly, physiologic reserve is reduced and the ability to maintain the physiology within the healthy is blunted. Take, for example, elderly patients and the ability to adapt to a salt load delivered by dietary means or the health care system. This process primarily involves both cardiac and renal adaptation. Studies reveal that healthy older adults have "stiffer" hearts and, therefore, do not achieve as much increased cardiac output induced by ventricular stretch and Starling curve with this volume expansion. Just as important, even in healthy older kidneys, salt excretion occurs less efficiently and takes longer. This lowered threshold for maintaining homeostasis, coined homeostenosis, results from a decreased ability of the systems built to interact with and modulate such deviations from physiologic normal. Another example of this involves changes in the autonomic nervous system. Changes in receptor sensitivity and feedback-loop automaticity result in a loss of variation in heart-rate response to stimuli. In the salt-load example, even in the normal healthy older adult, the ability to increase heart rate is limited and impedes the cardiorenal system from filtering salt as rapidly as in younger adults. One can discern from these examples that in describing systemic physiologic changes it becomes difficult to isolate each system or organ, because of how they work together and respond to one another while adjusting and adapting to carry out daily functions. The next section explores more specifically the relationship between known normative age-related changes in physiology and their impact on oral health.

SYSTEMIC CHANGES ASSOCIATED WITH ORAL HEALTH
Cardiovascular

Normal cardiovascular changes with age are both structural and functional. There is an overall decreased cardiovascular reserve with a loss of and hypertrophy of myocytes; 90% of pacemaker cells in the sinus node are lost by the age of 75 years,[1] resulting in slower resting and maximum heart rates. As described by Cefalu,[1] normal aging increases stiffness of the left ventricle, resulting in a decrease in left ventricular compliance. Even with the addition of left ventricular filling resulting in atrial contraction, the normal aged left ventricle creates a higher left ventricular end-diastolic pressure, a more robust Starling curve position point, and a higher stroke volume as the ventricle moves from diastole to systole. Arterial stiffness, the result of age-related calcification and collagen deposition in place of elastin, coupled with vasodilatory effects of decreased nitrous oxide, raises systolic vascular resistance, further impeding forward flow, increasing myocardial oxygen demand, and increasing cardiac work. In addition to the aforementioned normative changes in left ventricular function, the aging heart experiences decreasing abilities to raise the heart rate and has more muted responses to cholinergic and sympathomimetic stimulation, thus limiting the heart's ability to respond to additional stress including, but not limited to, exercise. This process results in an increased risk of congestive heart failure or heart block in the presence of chronic disease processes such as diabetes, hypertension, and coronary heart disease. Despite these changes the cardiovascular system compensates to maintain function, but finds it is difficult to adapt during stress or a medical intervention such as a dental appointment.[2]

In the dental office, this can translate clinically to understanding the changes in blood pressure found in older adults. With the normal aging heart blood pressure tends to increase, partially because of decreased compliance of the aorta and flexibility in the arteries. Systolic pressure has been known to continuously increase with age whereas diastolic pressure fluctuates with age, leading to an increase in pulse pressure. In adults older than 50 years, increased pulse pressure and systolic blood pressure greater than 140 mm Hg is a more significant risk factor for heart disease than diastolic blood pressure.[3,4] Hypertension, a risk factor for cardiovascular disease and one of the most common medical conditions among older adults, affects approximately two-thirds and three-fourths of men and women, respectively, older than 75 years.[5] As a result of aforementioned physiologic changes with aging, clinicians are now more concerned about hypertension defined as systolic blood pressure greater than 160 mm Hg than with the conventional definition of hypertension, blood pressure greater than 140/90 mm Hg.[5] In addition, because of blunted baroreceptors in the carotid arteries that do not modulate acute changes in blood pressure in normal aging, oral health providers must also be aware of postural hypotension likely to occur in normal individuals on standing from a sitting or lying position in the dental chair.[1]

Pulmonary

Normal structural changes with age in the respiratory system include: stiffening of the rib cage; reduced diaphragmatic and intercostal muscle strength, including early fatigue of the diaphragm; decreased chemoreceptive response (reducing the perception of dyspnea); alterations in connective tissue; reduced airway size and shallower alveolar cells and sacs; and decreased vital capacity and forced expiratory volume, with an increase in residual volume and functional residual capacity.[1] Although all of these physiologic changes are considered normal and continue to maintain respiration, they lower the threshold for adaptive ability, increase the risk of disease, and have an effect on oral health.

Many of these changes contribute to a decreased cough reflex and defective mucus clearance, directly affecting oral health through an increase the risk of aspiration both in the dental chair during treatment and through plaque accumulation on teeth and dentures.[6] In addition, normative changes with age associated with decreased genioglossal reflex and an elongated soft palate increase the risk for obstructive sleep apnea (OSA) and hypertension secondary to OSA.

Musculoskeletal

In the normal aging process of the musculoskeletal system, there is a decline in bone mineralization and architectural strength of the boney matrices. Microfractures accumulate and joints stiffen as a result of a decline in water content in the tendons, ligaments, cartilage, and synovial compartment.[1] In addition, both muscle mass and total body water decrease with an increase in total body fat. This process increases the distribution of water-soluble medications such as acetaminophen, effectively concentrating the dose in older adults in comparison with younger adults. Conversely, the distribution of lipid-soluble medications decreases, and drugs such as diazepam and lidocaine (commonly administered by dentists) have a longer half-life owing to their distribution throughout adipose tissue.[7]

Normal age-related functional changes may also include reduction in hand-grip strength, with a greater loss in the lower extremities than in the upper extremities.[1] In healthy but frailer individuals, this could affect tooth brushing and flossing efficiency. Toothbrush modifications may need to be made to accommodate an individual's ability.

Liver

As the liver ages it decreases in size by approximately 1% every year beginning at age 40 years, and as the aging process continues blood flow to the liver decreases by 40% to 45%.[7] In vivo and in vitro studies have also shown a decrease in hepatic metabolic activity, further reducing liver function with age.[8] These changes affect hepatic drug metabolism and clearance, and should be taken into consideration when prescribing medications.

Kidney

The normal aging kidney undergoes structural and physiologic changes that may compromise functional reserve, such as a decrease in glomerular and tubular mass, a decrease in glomerular filtration rate (GFR; a measurement of renal function), and decreased renal blood flow. By age 40 years, the GFR declines by a rate of 1% per year. Even with these changes, the healthy kidney maintains homeostasis of body fluids. In older adults with and without chronic kidney disease, renal excretion of medications takes longer than in younger adults.[1,7,9]

The clinical importance in dentistry of such age-related physiologic changes is linked with prescribing medication and scheduling of appointments. Classes of drugs commonly prescribed by dentists for which changes in dosed medication are important to prevent side effects include fluoroquinolones (phototoxicity, hallucinations, delusions, seizures, cognitive dysfunction), penicillins (seizures, cognitive dysfunction), fluconazole, and aminoglycoside antibiotics.[1,10]

Owing to the diminished physiologic reserve of both the liver and the kidney associated with the aging process and possible comorbidities, the body's ability to respond to external stress decreases. To decrease potential external stress, it is important to take into consideration appointment time, duration, and procedure type when scheduling elderly patients.

ORAL AND PHARYNGEAL CHANGES

The normal aging process of adults encompasses many physiologic changes in the oral cavity; however, many of these changes are secondary to chronic systemic disease and their treatment regimens (medication, chemotherapy, radiotherapy).[11] This section focuses on the normative changes in the aging oral cavity rather than the pathologic changes associated with disease.

Dentition

As described earlier, distinguishing from normal changes and abnormal changes in aging is challenging, and often differs from person to person. The aging of dentition is no different, and involves several changes accumulated over time depending on mechanical and chemical wear from mastication, in addition to factors such as culture, diet, occupation, tooth composition and resiliency, and the strength of teeth and surrounding periodontal apparatus.[12]

Enamel

Enamel is the hardest tissue in the human body, composed of 93% hydroxyapatite, 2% to 3% water, 2% carbonate, and trace amounts of sodium, magnesium, potassium, chloride, zinc, lipids, and fluoride primarily functioning to protect the tooth.[13] Despite the broad spectrum of changes that occur in aging dentition, is has been observed that changes occur in both physical appearance and molecular composition in healthy aging adults. Beginning early in life on eruption of the anterior permanent incisors, mamelons (small enamel protuberances along the incisal edge) are usually worn off completely; and occlusal wear continues throughout life. Enamel has the greatest content of mineralization in the human body. A study in 2008 found the elastic modulus and hardness of the outer enamel surface to increase by 16% and 12%, respectively, in old enamel when compared with young enamel.[14] Because of these molecular changes it is likely that teeth are more brittle and less permeable, contributing to cracks and microfractures in tooth enamel in aging teeth.[12] As a lifetime of normal occlusal wear develops, it can be difficult to distinguish between normal and pathologic tooth wear. Bruxism and clenching, 2 significant oral problems in aging adults, can exacerbate normal occlusal wear and contribute to parafunctional habits, leading to pain and complex (and potentially expensive) treatment options.[15]

Dentin

Lying just below enamel, dentin consists of 70% mineral hydroxyapatite by weight, of which 20% is organic material and 10% is water. Two major structural changes that occur with age are the formation of both physiologic and reparative secondary dentin and sclerosis of the dentinal tubules, resulting in decreased sensation to cold, hot, sweet, and pain. It is possible that at age 80 years, most of the dentinal tubules have been fully occluded.[12] It has also been reported that dentin undergoes a reduction in fracture toughness depending on age, contributing to mechanical changes related to age.[16]

Pulp

Dental pulp consists of highly vascularized and innervated connective tissue whose primary response to stimulus is pain. In addition to normative changes to aging enamel and dentin, it has been found that normal histologic changes to aging pulpal tissue decrease the pulpal response to stimuli.[17] It is common that older adults will not complain of tooth pain from occlusal wear, rampant decay, infection, or inflammation, and that disease will go unnoticed and unreported. A study conducted by Farac and colleagues[17] of adults older than 60 years confirms that pulp response time increases with age because of increased collagenous fibers and calcification, decreased blood supply, and nerve fiber degeneration. From a questionnaire distributed to endodontists in 2001, Goodis and colleagues[18] found that most diplomates surveyed agreed that the root canal decreases in size with age, supporting evidence reporting a narrowing of the pulpal chamber attributable to secondary and tertiary dentin formation, increased connective tissue within the pulp, and decreased innervation and vascularization.[18] In addition, through research conducted by Kress and colleagues,[19] lower signal intensity through high-powered magnetic resonance imaging examination was found to be age-dependent. This finding further demonstrates age-dependent changes to the pulp caused by increased deposition of dentin.

Cementum

Cementum lines the root surface connecting the tooth to the periodontium. As cementum ages its thickness increases 3-fold between the ages of 10 and 75 years, with the thickest layer at the apex and varying degrees of thickness along the root depending on recession and wear of the root surface.[12]

Changes that occur in the structures of the tooth contribute to decreased sensitivity to thermal conduction and reporting of pain. Fewer older adults report tooth pain attributable to molecular changes in enamel, dentin, pulpal tissue, and cementum. **Figs. 1** and **2** illustrate some of the physiologic changes that take place within these structures.

Periodontal Apparatus

It is thought that minimal loss of alveolar bone and the periodontal attachment apparatus is common in older adults, not as a consequence of aging but of the disease process.

Epidemiologic studies show a higher prevalence of periodontal disease in older cohorts than in younger cohorts, most likely attributable to cumulative tissue destruction over a lifetime rather than an age-dependent risk of periodontal susceptibility.[20–22]

Oral Mucosa

The function of the oral mucosa is to provide a host defense, mastication, swallowing, speech, and flavor perception.[11] Although it has been reported that during the normal

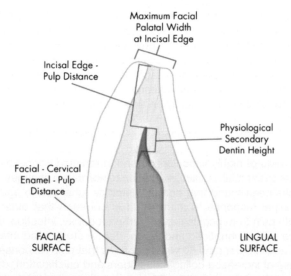

Fig. 1. Increases with age of physiologic secondary dentin height and incisal edge enamel-pulp distance. (*Courtesy of* Gregory An, DDS, MPH.)

YOUNG TOOTH   OLD TOOTH

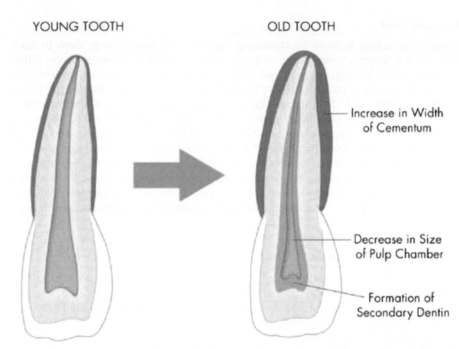

Increase in Width
of Cementum

Decrease in Size
of Pulp Chamber

Formation of
Secondary Dentin

Fig. 2. Changes to dentin with aging. The secondary dentin grows inwardly into the pulp chamber, decreasing the chamber's size. (*Courtesy of* Gregory An, DDS, MPH.)

aging process the oral mucosa thins, loses elasticity, and has a diminished attachment to underlying bone and connective tissue, there is a paucity of data on this subject, making it difficult to interpret the results.[1,23] An emphasis on research on changes in oral mucosa secondary to disease, medication use, and radiation and chemotherapy has provided clinicians with possible diagnoses and treatment options to ameliorate the symptoms.

Saliva

Saliva is vital to maintaining oropharyngeal health and function by aiding in speech, taste, digestion, swallowing, and oral cleansing. Without its lubricating and antimicrobial effects, oral and extraoral disorders are more prevalent, including discomfort.[24] Dry mouth is a common complaint among approximately 30% of older adults; however, it is not a part of normal aging.[25] Results from the Baltimore Longitudinal Study of Aging in 1988 reported no age-related change in salivary flow rates of stimulated parotid and stimulated and unstimulated submandibular glands.[26] In another study by Baum[27] examining healthy adults aged 22 to 88 years taking no medications, stimulated parotid saliva was examined and was found to have no diminished fluid output. While it has long been known that salivary function is relatively age-independent, it continues to be shown that salivary output does not change with age in healthy older adults. Data on salivary composition of electrolytes and proteins, however, varies even among healthy adults.[10,23,24] The primary reason for reported change in salivary function is that it occurs secondary to disease or treatment modalities.

Self-induced dehydration manifesting as a fear of toileting or a lack of thirst is common in the elderly and can affect salivary flow, deglutition, and interest in eating.[28]

Taste and Smell

Saliva plays a role in taste by dissolving tastants and transporting them to taste buds on the tongue, palate, and/or oropharynx. The tastes of sweet, sour, bitter, salt, and umami (savory) are detected and buffered by different salivary constituents such as salivary bicarbonate, salivary carbonate, and salivary glutamate, and play a role in host defense.[11] Tylenda and Baum[26] found there to be no age difference in detection of intensity of 2 taste qualities in nonmedicated individuals. There is a paucity of recent data, however, on taste perception in aging adults and on the aging effect on taste buds and taste. Regarding the tongue, results of aging studies on the number or density of taste buds present in the aging adult are contradictory, while results from a study by Kano and colleagues[29] showed a significant decrease in the mean density of taste buds on the laryngeal surface of the epiglottis. Although gustation is relatively unaffected, olfaction undergoes significant age-related changes.[11,26]

Mastication, Speech, and Swallowing

Altered mastication has been one of the most reported oral motor disturbances in older adults.[30] Few studies have reported specifically on masticatory muscles changes with aging; however, reduced cross-sectional area, reduced muscle density, twitch prolongation, and diminished strength (tongue and masticatory muscles) have been reported. Such changes could be due to loss of muscle fibers or muscle fiber atrophy, or both. In addition, those without teeth were found to have greater decreases in area than those with teeth. The ability for individuals to masticate has an impact on food preferences and perceived taste, texture, and ease of chewing,[30] further affecting the nutrition, systemic health, and quality of life of older adults.

Swallowing is another oral motor function requiring the coordination of sufficient salivary flow, an intact mucosa, and neuromuscular processing to carry out the 3 phases of the swallowing process: oral, pharyngeal, and esophageal.[30] Normal changes found in the oropharynx include a lengthening of the soft palate, more significant in women than in men. In both sexes, the parapharyngeal tissues experience an increase in the fat pad, independent of body mass index. In addition, physiologic changes in the genioglossal response to negative pressure in the pharynx, mimicking other upper airway muscle responses to pressure changes, reduce pharyngeal patency, and decrease the threshold for collapse of the upper airway and pharynx. Recent data suggest that despite changes in the normal aging process, its impact on swallowing is subtle and clinically insignificant.[30] Difficulty in swallowing increases the risk of choking/aspiration, and may result from decreased salivary production on taking medications, cerebrovascular and neurologic disorders, arthritis, diabetes, pulmonary diseases, and a decreased number of teeth with which to masticate, all of which may alter the speed, strength, and/or coordination of the musculature.[30]

Speech is an oral motor function with multiple components contributing to its function: tongue, sensory and motor innervation, salivary production, muscle tone and strength, respiration, and vertical dimension of occlusion. All of these components affect speech and as they age with time so does their function and, consequently, that of speech.[23] That being said, speech is not significantly altered during the normal aging process. Common age-related changes in speech may be a slowed speaking rate, an increase in pauses, and inaccurate articulation. None of these conditions, however, are considered disorders; systemic diseases such as Parkinson disease or cerebrovascular accidents can lead to speech impairments.[30]

SUMMARY

Oral health plays a vital role in several functions that contribute to quality of life, longevity, and functional independence. The oral cavity, when functioning properly, provides and contributes to: the enjoyment of taste; smell; the appropriate steps needed for deglutition and swallowing; nutrition; maintenance of facial anatomy; and self-esteem. This article focuses on the normative changes in health relative to oral health in aging adults. The age-related changes discussed are independent of disease or medication use, and are essential in understanding how these physiologic changes contribute to a lower threshold for developing disease. A decreased physiologic reserve with normal age-related changes in health coupled with decreased access to care can be more difficult to cope with for an older adult in comparison with younger counterparts. Older adults also differ more from one another physiologically than younger adults, which makes geriatric care a greater challenge for the clinician.

REFERENCES

1. Cefalu C. Theories and mechanisms of aging. Clin Geriatr Med 2011;27:491–506.
2. Bergman SA, Coletti D. Perioperative management of the geriatric patient. Part II: cardiovascular system. Oral Surg Oral Med Oral Pathol Oral Radiol Endod 2006; 102:e7–12.
3. Glick M. The new blood pressure guidelines. J Am Dent Assoc 2004;135:585–6.
4. Pinto E. Blood pressure and ageing. Postgrad Med J 2007;83:109–14.
5. Lipsitz LA. A 91-year-old woman with difficult-to-control hypertension: a clinical review. JAMA 2013;310(12):1274–80.
6. Bergman SA, Coletti D. Perioperative management of the geriatric patient. Part I: respiratory system. Oral Surg Oral Med Oral Pathol Oral Radiol Endod 2006;102: e1–6.
7. Dental considerations for geriatric patients. Available at: http://www.netce.com/ 839/Course_3956.pdf.
8. Zeeh J, Platt D. The aging liver: structural and functional changes and their consequences for drug treatment in old age. Gerontology 2002;48:121–7.
9. Colloca G, Santoro M, Gambassi G. Age-related physiologic changes and perioperative management of elderly patients. Surg Oncol 2010;19:124–30.
10. Mangoni AA, Jackson SH. Age-related changes in pharmacokinetics and pharmacodynamics: basic principles and practical applications. Br J Clin Pharmacol 2004;57(1):6–14.
11. Ship JA. The influence of aging on oral health and consequences for taste and smell. Physiol Behav 1999;66(2):209–15.
12. An G. Normal aging of teeth. Geriatr Aging 2009;12(10):513–7.
13. Garcia-Godoy F, Hicks MJ. Maintaining the integrity of the enamel surface: the role of dental biofilm, saliva, and preventative agents in enamel demineralization and remineralization. J Am Dent Assoc 2008;139(Suppl 2):25S–34S.
14. Park S, Wang DH, Zhang D, et al. Mechanical properties of human enamel as a function of age and location in the tooth. J Mater Sci Mater Med 2008;19: 2317–24.
15. Christensen GJ. Providing oral care for the aging patient. J Am Dent Assoc 2007; 138:239–42.
16. Lund AE. Dentin grows more brittle with age. J Am Dent Assoc 2009;140(12): 1472.
17. Farac RV, Morgental RD, de Pontes Lima RK, et al. Pulp sensibility test in elderly patients. Gerodontology 2012;29:135–9.

18. Goodis HE, Rossall JC, Kahn AJ. Endodontic status in older U.S. adults. J Am Dent Assoc 2001;132:1525–30.
19. Kress B, Buhl Y, Hahnel S, et al. Age- and tooth-related pulp cavity signal changes in healthy teeth: a comparative magnetic resonance imaging analysis. Oral Surg Oral Med Oral Pathol Oral Radiol Endod 2007;103(1):134–7.
20. Boehm TK, Scannapieco FA. The epidemiology, consequences and management of periodontal disease in older adults. J Am Dent Assoc 2007;138(Suppl 9):26S–33S.
21. Douglass CW. Risk assessment and management of periodontal disease. J Am Dent Assoc 2006;137(Suppl 3):27S–32S.
22. Timmerman MF, van der Weijden GA. Risk factors for periodontitis. Int J Dent Hyg 2006;4(1):2–7.
23. Sonies BC, Stone M, Shawker T. Speech and swallowing in the elderly. Gerodontology 1984;3(2):115–23.
24. Turner MD, Ship JA. Dry mouth and its effects on the oral health of elderly. J Am Dent Assoc 2007;138(Suppl 1):15S–20S.
25. Berkey DB, Scannapieco FA. Medical considerations relating to the oral health of older adults. Spec Care Dentist 2013;33(4):164–76.
26. Tylenda CA, Baum BJ. Oral physiology and the Baltimore longitudinal study of aging. Gerodontology 1988;7(1):5–9.
27. Baum BJ. Evaluation of stimulated parotid saliva flow rate in different age groups. J Dent Res 1981;60(7):1292–6.
28. National Institute of Aging. Go 4 life: drinking enough fluid. Available at: http://go4life.nia.nih.gov/sites/default/flles/DrinkingEnoughFluids.pdf.
29. Kano M, Shimizu Y, Okayama K, et al. Quantitative study of ageing epiglottal taste buds in humans. Gerodontology 2007;24:169–72.
30. Chavez EM, Ship JA. Sensory and motor deficits in the elderly: impact on oral health. J Public Health Dent 2000;60(4):297–303.

Treatment Planning Considerations in Older Adults

Ella M. Oong, DMD, MPH, Gregory K. An, DDS, MPH*

KEYWORDS

- Treatment planning • Geriatric • Decision making • Informed consent • Dental
- Oral health • Older adults • Elderly

KEY POINTS

- Treatment planning for geriatric care is a dynamically informed process culminating from comprehensive diagnostic evaluation and informed consent.
- Geriatric patients presenting with multiple chronic conditions, medications, and complex sociobehavioral histories require a strategic, stepwise plan for disease treatment and oral health maintenance.
- Flexibility and good communication with the patient and other involved parties during treatment planning for older adults may attenuate uncertainties and lead to successful outcomes.

INTRODUCTION

Treatment planning in a healthy, older adult is usually straightforward, varying little from the process clinicians typically follow. Normal changes in the aging dentition can require very little modification to the usual treatment-planning process. Often, though, developing dental treatment plans for older adults is complicated by their declining status in general health, cognitive function, and functional ability.

This article briefly describes the profile of older adults in the United States, and discusses the dynamic process of treatment planning and obtaining informed consent. Next, various models for formulating alternative treatment plans are described. Finally, a case is presented that illustrates treatment planning for multiple chronic conditions and polypharmacy.

Funding Sources: None.
Conflict of Interest: None.
Private Practice, 1690 Woodside Road, Suite 209, Redwood City, CA 94061, USA
* Corresponding author.
E-mail address: gregan@post.harvard.edu

PROFILE OF OLDER ADULTS

Thirteen percent of the United States population is 65 years and older, with the young-old (age 65–74 years) comprising 7%, the old (age 75–84) 4%, and the old-old (age ≥85) 2%.[1] In large part because of the shift away from infectious diseases as the leading causes of death, Americans are living longer than ever before. In 1960, at birth Americans were expected to live 69.7 years; today they are expected to live at least 78 years. With a declining birth rate, the first group of baby-boomers reaching 65, and the increasing life expectancy, the United States is developing into an aging society (**Fig. 1**).[2,3] The life expectancy in 1960 for people age 65 was 14.3 years. Half a century later, life expectancy for older adults has increased to 19.1 years.

Although most people 65 years and older live in the community, only 3% at any given time live in a skilled nursing facility (SNF).[4] However, the percentage of elderly living in SNFs increases with age; in 2010, less than 1% of the young-old and 13.5% of the old-old lived in an SNF. In addition to being older, residents living in these facilities tend to be sicker and more functionally impaired.[5] An increasing need for long-term care combined with shortages in the workforce and physical space in nursing homes shifts the burden of disease toward the community at large.[6] Almost 20% of community-dwelling older adults suffer from a psychiatric disorder[7] while approximately 28% of older adults have 3 or more chronic diseases.[8] From 2007 to 2010, 89% of those aged 65 and older took at least one prescription drug in past 30 days, and 66.6% took 3 or more prescription drugs.[9] Despite improvement in maintaining functional status, in 2010 23% of older adults had at least one basic action difficulty or complex activity limitation.[3,9] Those persons most functionally impaired with loss of activities of daily living (ADLs) are increasing in proportion.[10] With an aging population, oral health needs, which can affect quality of life and overall health, remain a concern.

As the United States increasingly ages, older adults have retained more teeth than ever before. In 1965, every other man or woman older than 65 years in the United States had no natural teeth.[11] By contrast, in 2002 fewer than 25% of older adults were edentulous.[12] However, older adults with a chronic condition such as diabetes, arthritis, cardiovascular disease, or chronic obstructive pulmonary disease, experienced a higher rate of tooth loss and edentulism than those without a condition.[13] Furthermore, increasing numbers of elderly still necessitates fixed and removable complete dentures (CDs).[14] Sixty-four percent of older adults have either moderate or severe periodontitis.[15] Approximately 1 in 5 older adults have untreated coronal caries[13,16]; similarly, 1 in 5 report xerostomia.[17] Twelve percent of adults age 60 years and older have root caries.[12] The need for treatment exists.

In recognition of treatment needs, older adults continue to seek dental care. From 2000 to 2011, dental utilization among older adults increased from 38% to 42% (Medical Expenditure Panel Survey[18]). This trend is consistent with previous analyses of the same survey, which showed greater utilization among older adults than younger adults.[19] In 2007, 92% of dentists report treating vulnerable elderly patients.[20] In the same survey, dentists indicate a lack of information about managing patients with complex medical histories, xerostomia, and dementia. In the next sections, management of the treatment-planning process for older patients is discussed.

GOALS OF THE TREATMENT-PLANNING PROCESS

Treatment planning is the culmination of a comprehensive diagnostic process that usually precedes routine treatment.[21,22] A goal of treatment planning should be the development of a systematic means of action to eradicate dental disease, reestablish

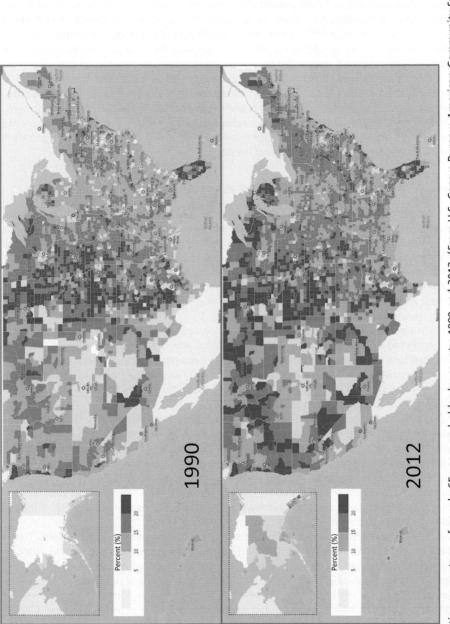

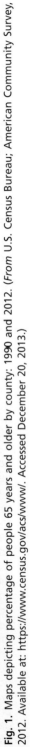

Fig. 1. Maps depicting percentage of people 65 years and older by county: 1990 and 2012. (*From* U.S. Census Bureau; American Community Survey, 2012. Available at: https://www.census.gov/acs/www/. Accessed December 20, 2013.)

and preserve as much function as possible, and enhance quality of life.[21,23] It should address the underlying disease process giving rise to signs and symptoms found on examination and elicited from patients.[22,24] Treatment plans should also attend to patients' chief complaints as quickly as possible, rely on individual needs, and prevent and manage tooth loss.[25,26] Furthermore, treatment plans should communicate the role of caregivers in maintenance and care, account for realistic circumstances, be continuously informed, make dental appointments as comfortable as possible, and emphasize continued monitoring of oral health and a functional dentition.[27] The most influential factors in comprehensive treatment planning are patients' disease status, followed by patients' requests, and lastly, patients' ability to pay.[21] The treatment-planning process facilitates diagnosis of disease(s) and results in a plan that accounts for patients' interests and expectations, treats diagnosed problems, and provides a stepwise strategy for maintaining oral health.

REVIEW OF CONVENTIONAL TREATMENT PLANNING

Treatment plans vary in the breadth of services required and the degree of comprehensiveness involved in treatment delivered. The simplest treatment plan consists of no treatment. On another level, limited treatment plans address only emergency and/or palliative care. Basic treatment plans are expanded in scope by providing for additional procedures such as scaling and root planing, denture relines, or minor operative interventions. Comprehensive treatment plans inherently address more complicated, multistep, sequenced procedures, which usually entail different disciplines such as endodontics and prosthodontics (**Fig. 2**).

With regard to comprehensive treatment planning, treatment considerations are incorporated through several phases dynamically informed by patient desires. Comprehensive treatment, as outlined in the treatment plan, is accomplished over these phases: diagnostic evaluation phase, priority and acute phase, disease control phase, restorative phase subdivided into preprosthetic and definitive prosthetic, and maintenance and prevention phase.[28]

Diagnosis of disease and resultant treatment plans culminate from a thorough diagnostic evaluation that assembles the following information: complete medical history, patient information and chief complaint, history of present illness, dental history, social history, family history, review of systems, intraoral/extraoral examination, laboratory results, vital signs, impressions and models, imaging such as radiographs, and photographs.[22,28] Additional information is often retrieved by a consultation with the patient's physician; the consultation may require follow-up conversations with multiple care providers in cases with a complicated medical history.[29]

Acute issues of an emergent or palliative nature are immediately addressed. Treatment of acute pain exemplifies a pressing issue requiring immediate attention. After an emergency or palliative phase, a disease-control component manages any extended conditions such as initial periodontal treatment, caries control activities, and prevention activities. The restorative and aesthetics phase following disease control may be further subdivided into a preprosthetic phase and definitive prosthetic phase. Critical sequencing in preparation for final restorations is planned during this phase. The preprosthetic phase often entails advanced treatment in oral surgery, endodontics, orthodontics, periodontal surgery, and implant placement. The final prosthetic phase involves certain types of permanent operative restorations, fixed and removable final prostheses. Finally, in the maintenance and prevention phase, all treatment is reevaluated and the patient is placed on a maintenance schedule. An appropriate prevention plan for the time interval between recall examinations is also determined.

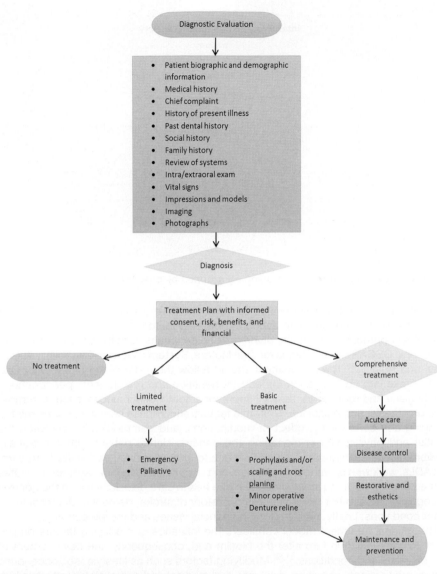

Fig. 2. Conventional treatment-planning process.

MODELS OF GERIATRIC DENTAL TREATMENT PLANNING

This section provides an overview of treatment-planning models that attempt to account for the myriad of considerations accompanying dental care for the elderly, and **Fig. 3** presents a diagram summarizing of the factors presented in these models. A straightforward yet comprehensive approach to treatment planning for older adults uses the familiar mnemonic SOAP (Subjective findings, Objective findings, Assessment, and Plan).[24] In geriatric patients, the subjective findings include additional information concerning functional status as described by the ability to carry out ADLs and instrumental activities of daily living.[24] Otherwise, objective findings and resultant assessment develop in the usual fashion. Finally, the plan section details any

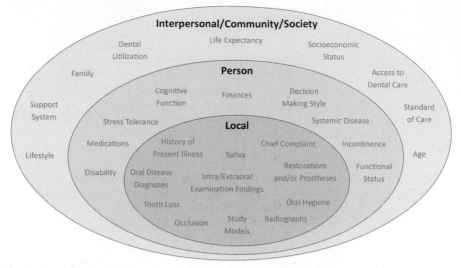

Fig. 3. Considerations in treatment planning grouped by proximity to oral health.

treatment performed and delineates a comprehensive, sequenced treatment plan, which may or may not take into account modifying factors.[22,24]

Another approach to treatment planning for older adults uses the easy to remember mnemonic OSCAR, which stands for Oral factors, Systemic factors, Capability, Autonomy, and Reality.[30] The assessment should follow the order of the mnemonic. Oral factors take into consideration the current dentition and restorations, periodontium, oral hygiene and root caries, salivary secretions, tooth loss, mucosal tissues, removable prosthesis, and occlusion. Systemic factors encompass normal changes related to aging and comorbidity, effect of medications, and communication between the dentist and physician(s) in managing the geriatric dental patient with a medically compromised health status. Capability refers to attributes such as the ability to carry out ADLs, walk with or without assistance, and control incontinence. Autonomy relates to the patient's ability to independently make health care decisions within the context of cognitive impairment stemming from a history of stroke, dementia, depression, or other conditions. Lastly, reality refers to financial issues and life expectancy.

The rational treatment model considers the influence of modifying factors on primary factors, which in turn alter the biofilm and, consequently, the development of oral diseases and conditions.[31,32] Modifying factors such as lifestyle, socioeconomic status, medications, cognition, disability, and medical and dental history alter the balance of diet, saliva, and genetics, and affects chemotherapeutics and oral hygiene. This model, adapted from a caries risk model, explains how etiologic factors affect the development of caries, periodontal disease, tooth loss, and mucosal lesions. Furthermore, risks and benefits of treatment also influence whether no treatment, emergency care, limited treatment, or comprehensive care is planned. In addition, an example of the rational treatment model depicts the utility of a decision tree in treatment planning for dentate adults.[33] The patient's desires, expectations, dental needs, quality-of-life expectations, stress tolerance, financial status, and oral hygiene capacity, along with the dentist's experience and skill level, direct the treatment-planning process.[25,32]

Another model uses a clinical reasoning sequence in decision making and resolution of dental problems.[32] In the model, 3 action sequences are presented in resolving dental problems: (1) determine the cause, (2) choose an action, and (3) implement the plan. To determine cause, the problem must be defined, other possible causes considered, and possible causes tested. To help choose an action, goals in consultation with the patient must be established, alternatives examined, and adverse consequences considered. Finally, implementation of the plan involves anticipating potential problems, taking preventive actions, and setting up contingency plans. This systematic approach can be successful if the steps in the action sequences are effective.

Another approach addresses complexity and uncertainty in treatment planning in elderly patients, and provides a basis for prioritizing and weighing factors affecting the treatment-planning process.[34] More than 20 factors contribute to the process. Some important factors include: reliance on biological age rather than chronologic age; consideration of the useful life of dental interventions such as fillings and prosthetics in the context of life expectancy for older adults; and reconciliation of expectations between the patient, other involved parties, and the dentist through effective communication. To address uncertainties inherent to treatment planning, clear decisions should be made and treatment progress monitored. Careful documentation from evaluation to implementation protects from uncertainty.

Mulligan and Vanderlinde[35] present a geriatric care model that is intended to account for the factors precipitating successful treatment in any setting. The model depicts the interplay between 4 broad domains: dental/oral, medical, psychosocial, and behavioral. Examination findings, influence of systemic disease, physician consult, dental specialty referral, treatment plan modifications, and selection of appropriate treatment options constitute the factors within the dental/oral category. Suggested medical factors to consider include: systemic conditions; medications, including adverse effects and drug-drug interactions; laboratory values; special issues; and medical referral. Psychosocial factors influencing treatment plan include: informal assessment; basis of functioning such as cognition, recognition, reasoning, and commitment; and support system from the societal to the personal. Among behavioral factors, the areas of consideration are: decision-making style; ability to cooperate with treatment; sedation involving feasibility and need; understanding of one's own limitations; need for personal assistance; home-care capability; and adherence potential. This model guides the clinician in attenuating psychosocial, medical, and behavioral barriers.

Finally, a more specific approach to treatment planning addresses dementia and its role in planning.[27] In the early stage of dementia, when changes in cognitive function are minimal, changes to the treatment-planning process are minimal as well. However, if there is an accompanying degenerative disease diagnosis such as Alzheimer disease, the treatment plan should be designed to anticipate future loss of cognitive function, include aggressive prevention, and restore function with celerity. Treatment plans for middle and late stages of dementia may require considerations such as modifying appointment length, using sedation, and increasing the frequency of recalls. In the middle stages of dementia, it is suggested that limited treatment plans are designed with minimal changes, and should include aggressive prevention along with communication of prevention strategies with caregivers. Treatment of those at advanced and terminal stages may be basic, with palliative and emergency care aimed at maintaining the dentition. As described, many considerations are factored into treatment planning for the older adult. Nonetheless, throughout the treatment-planning process the patient's desires continually influence clinical decision making. However, communication between the dentist and an older patient can be complicated by competency and informed consent issues.

DECISION-MAKING CAPACITY, COMPETENCY, AND INFORMED CONSENT

Before any dental examination, the clinician must obtain a valid consent to treat or not treat. In general, informed consent requires a disclosure of the relevant risks of, benefits of, and alternatives to treatment that potentially affect the patient's decision on the treatment. However, proper disclosure by the clinician alone is insufficient to obtaining a valid consent. The patient must also possess decision-making capacity as defined by ability to comprehend, appreciate, and reason the contingencies of treatment or no treatment[36,37]; the ability to weigh the risks and benefits of treatment, no treatment, and alternatives; and the ability to communicate his or her choices.[37,38] In some instances, especially in the elderly, determination of capacity may be unclear and subject to bias.[36] The elderly with dementia and/or psychiatric illness, nursing home residents, and hospitalized elderly all have increased risk for reduced consent capacity.[39] In most cases when a patient is determined to lack capacity, the clinician assigns a health care proxy to consent for that patient. Dentists are legally bound by the same process and standards as physicians and other health care professionals in securing informed consent.[40] Therefore, dentists should know and comply with the legal obligation regarding capacity and informed consent for the state in which they practice.[41] The evaluation for capacity to consent for treatment should be a fluid process to be evaluated at each treatment decision. The patient should have self-determination of as much of their treatment as possible.

Although decision-making capacity and competency are similar; they are not synonymous. The legal determination of patient competency describes the ability of the patient to make informed decisions. However, patient competency differs in scope, determination, and purpose. Lack of capacity does not preclude a patient from making any decisions. Each decision varies in risk, benefits, and complexities, and should be independently assessed. When appropriate, patients should be empowered to make their own decisions. However, competency, formally determined by a court of law, concerns the individual's mental capacity to make autonomous decisions in general. At the time a person is determined incompetent, a court appoints a guardian who acts as a surrogate decision maker. In addition to health care decisions, the guardian handles decisions regarding contracts, finances, and other personal affairs. In this case, obtaining consent is straightforward; the guardian provides informed consent. A case is now presented that emphasizes many of the factors highlighted in this discussion of treatment-planning considerations.

AUTHORS' CASE REPORT
Presentation and Examination

A 73-year-old Greek American woman, Maria, was referred to our clinic by her internist. Her chief complaint was "I don't like the way my teeth look. It looks like I don't have teeth." She arrived with her 42-year-old niece. Maria suffered from osteoarthritis of the hips and knees, and had undergone total hip replacement on her right side 4 years ago. However, she still had some difficulty walking without the assistance of a cane. She was morbidly obese and experienced breathing difficulty on exertion. Maria's medical conditions and medications are listed in **Table 1**.

Maria immigrated to the United States from Greece as a teenager with her parents and one sister. She was a retired elementary school teacher, never had children, and lived alone with her 2 cats. At the time of treatment, Maria's sister and parents had been deceased. Her niece helped transport her to her medical and dental visits, and assisted with some daily chores. Her internist informed us Maria had intact ADL skills. Maria smoked cigarettes for more than 20 years and quit more than 10 years

Table 1
Medical status of the patient

Systemic Conditions	Mental Conditions	Medications
Arterial stents	Alzheimer disease	Baby aspirin
Chronic obstructive pulmonary disease	(stage 1: early/mild)	Citalopram
Coronary artery disease	Anxiety	Donepezil
Diabetes mellitus type 2	Depression	Hydrochlorothiazide
Hypercholesterolemia		Ibuprofen
Hypertension		Lisinopril
Mild rheumatoid arthritis in hands		Lorazepam
Obesity		Lovastatin
Osteoarthritis with previous total joint		Metformin
replacement		Warfarin

ago. She denied use of alcohol. At her initial appointment, Maria was verbally coherent. She occasionally forgot words but her communication skills remained largely intact. Her dementia was mild and she had clear decision-making capacity. Photographs and radiographs from her initial visit are presented in **Fig. 4**.

Maria strongly preferred not to be left without teeth at any point during treatment. She remarked on how as a child her friends and family complimented her on her beautiful smile. She expressed feelings of depression over her deteriorating appearance and inability to chew. She was edentulous on the maxilla and partially edentulous on the mandible. Her existing natural teeth consisted of her 6 mandibular anterior teeth and one mandibular first premolar on her right side (see **Fig. 4**B). Findings from her examination showed generalized periodontal attachment loss with slight mobility of all her teeth, periapical radiolucencies, extensive root caries, and recurrent decay under existing crowns (see **Fig. 4**C). Her existing maxillary CD exhibited poor upper lip support and a collapsed vertical dimension (see **Fig. 4**A, D). In addition, she showed signs of Kelly combination syndrome: bilateral increase of her maxillary tuberosities, canting of the occlusal plane upward toward the anterior, and loss of anterior alveolar ridge support (see **Fig. 4**E).[2] Maria informed us that the maxillary CD was more than 10 years old, and she never wore her mandibular removable partial denture (RPD) because of discomfort.

Factors in Assessment

An important part of assessment is identifying what the oral health problems are, how they formed, and why they are present. The processes of examining the oral cavity, diagnosing oral diseases, and identifying local factors that cause diseases may be routine for clinicians. However, more distal factors that contribute to oral health problems may be more difficult to identify; such factors include financial, psychosocial, and behavioral problems (see **Fig. 3**).[42,43]

The following are some examples from Maria's case. First, Maria lacked dental insurance for nearly a decade. She was on a fixed income and thought that dental care was "too expensive." She sparingly visited the dentist and did not perceive any need. She only came to see us after her geriatrician made the referral when she complained about the appearance of her smile. Maria did not realize that her oral health was in decline, because of her lack of symptoms and perceived needs. Second, Maria's depression and anxiety likely negatively affected her hygiene habits, diet, oral health perception, and motivation.[44,45] Depressed elders are less likely to be interested in oral hygiene and more likely to consume a cariogenic diet.[46,47] A third example is the possible effects on Maria's oral health by her diabetes; diabetes, especially

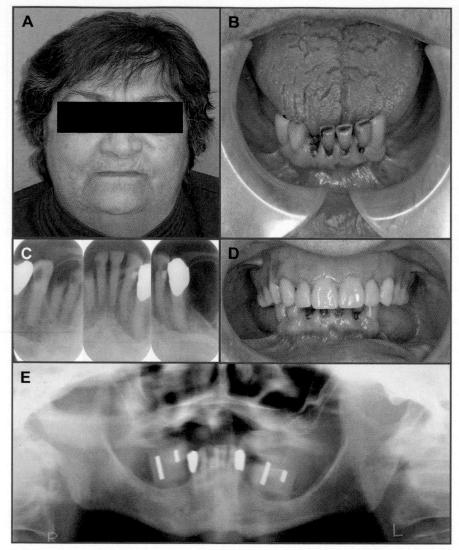

Fig. 4. Pretreatment photos and radiographs. (*A*) Face showing lack of lip support. (*B*) Remaining teeth. (*C*) Periapical radiographs. (*D*) Preexisting maxillary complete denture. (*E*) Panoramic radiograph.

when uncontrolled, has been identified as a risk factor for several diseases such as periodontal disease, caries, and endodontic infections.[47–50] Fourth, the link between cardiovascular disease and periodontal disease has been well documented, with nearly 500 peer-reviewed articles on the subject published between 1950 and 2011.[51] Maria's coronary artery disease (CAD) may have been associated with her periodontal disease and partial edentulism. Moreover, a history of periodontal disease may have contributed to her missing teeth. Finally, a side effect of nearly all of her medications is xerostomia. Xerostomia has been well documented to cause multiple oral health problems such as the root surface caries and periodontal disease that were observed in Maria's mouth.[52] For a more detailed discussion about the effects of systemic diseases and medications on oral health, please refer to the article by Tavares and colleagues on systemic and oral health elsewhere in this issue. As demonstrated, the combination of Maria's lack of perceived need, financial barrier, comorbidities, and polypharmacy are likely to have contributed to the decline in her oral health.

Factors in Planning and Implementation

At first glance, Maria's primary complaint may indicate a straightforward denture remake. However, after gathering more information, several factors arise that add complexity to the planning and implementing process. Her multiple chronic conditions may limit her tolerance for treatment and increase likelihood for fragmented and multi-provider medical care.[53] Moreover, the effects of her numerous medications would necessitate modifying her dental treatment. The following are several examples of how these factors influence treatment.

First, Maria's progressing Alzheimer disease may warrant a more aggressive treat-ment approach in anticipation of decline.[27] For example, early extractions and implants may be good options. Second, if a removable prosthesis is planned, it should be designed for easy removal because of the rheumatoid arthritis in her hands, yet it should still be retentive and stable in the mouth, enabling her to chew, speak, and smile. Third, one should consider having Maria sit upright for dental treatment because of breathing difficulties exacerbated by her chronic obstructive pulmonary disease (COPD) when lying supine. Fourth, epinephrine in local anesthetics should be limited to 0.036 mg per visit because of Maria's CAD.[54,55] Moreover, short appointments later in the morning are recommended for patients with cardiovascular disease.[54,56] Fifth, arterial stents do not require antibiotic prophylaxis[57]; however, as of this publication date, antibiotic prophylaxis before certain dental procedures may be required for pa-tients with total joint replacement beyond the previously recommended period of 2 years after replacement.[58] A consult with the patient's orthopedic surgeon is recom-mended. Details for joint replacement antibiotic prophylaxis recommendations are discussed in an article by Tavares and colleagues elsewhere in this issue. Sixth, Ma-ria's xerostomia and COPD increase her risk for dysphagia and aspiration pneu-monia.[59,60] Treatment modifications such as nonalcoholic chlorhexidine treatment, fluoride treatment, frequent recall, or, in the extreme case, extractions may help to reduce the presence of bacteria and plaque in the mouth.[52,61,62] Lastly, Maria's inter-nist or cardiologist should be consulted to manage her anticoagulation medications during her dental treatment. For invasive procedures such as extractions, implants, and periodontal and endodontic surgeries, the international normalized ratio (INR) should ideally be recorded on the day of surgery and no more than 48 hours before surgery.[63] Most instances of dental surgery will not require cessation of warfarin ther-apy if the INR is kept below 4.0.[64] If the INR is near the higher range, the dentist should be prepared to manage bleeding peri-/postoperatively. Moreover, when a patient like Maria is on multiple anticoagulant medications, it may be necessary to stop 1 or more of the medications before surgery. These examples illustrate a few of the management considerations that must take place during treatment in a patient presenting with mul-tiple chronic conditions and medications.

Treatment

A challenging component of planning for Maria's treatment and that for other elders, especially those who are frail, is the uncertainty with prognosis and outcomes of the various treatment modalities resulting from multiple influencing variables and the lack of good evidence. Therefore, development of a rational treatment plan becomes a subjective process biased by a clinician's experience.[1] Maria's case is no different. The treatment presented herein is one of several rational treatment options that could have effectively addressed her chief complaint and dental needs.

Maria wanted more natural-looking teeth but also wanted to be able to chew her food and speak without her dentures "flopping around." Although she presented with multiple chronic conditions, Maria was functioning highly with intact ADLs at the start of her treatment. She could tolerate most dental procedures including endodontic and implant procedures. However, cost was a major limiting factor for Maria and she had no desire to have fixed prosthetics. Therefore, we considered removable prosthetic options that would meet her aesthetic and functional needs in consideration of her limited financial resources, physical limitations, and impending disease progression.

Her remaining 7 mandibular teeth were extracted. Antibiotic prophylaxis was administered before surgery on the orthopedic surgeon's recommendation. During the same extraction surgery, 2 implants were immediately placed in the mandibular canine regions to serve as overdenture abutments. Thus we avoided separate surgeries for each procedure. Immediate maxillary and mandibular CDs were fabricated before surgery (**Fig. 5**A, B) and delivered immediately afterward (see **Fig. 5**D). After discussion with her cardiologist, we maintained warfarin treatment but stopped aspirin 10 days before surgery. Her INR was identified to be 2.8 at 4 hours before surgery with a quick capillary finger-stick test. Bleeding was well controlled during and after surgery with hemostatic techniques and good suturing (see **Fig. 5**C).

Alternative Treatment Comparisons

An alternative to extractions would have been to undergo caries control, endodontic and periodontal treatment, and crowns. Aesthetic correction would be much more challenging if mandibular teeth were left in place. For example, **Fig. 5**A, B shows the wax-up of the immediate CDs and illustrates the excessive overjet present.

In Maria's case the benefits of implants outweighed attempting to restore her teeth: there was a significant cost saving; implant abutments would be much easier to maintain as her dementia would lead to increased disability and frailty; the prognosis for the alternative endodontic and periodontal treatment may be worsened by her comorbidities[47–50]; her risk for dental decay for the future would be eliminated; and the simultaneous fabrication of the maxillary and mandibular CDs allowed for an immediate improvement in aesthetics. Implant-supported mandibular overdenture has become the standard of care for completely edentulous patients.[65,66] Moreover, improvements in oral health–related quality of life have been well documented.[67–69] However, the evidence comparing mandibular RPDs and implant-supported overdentures is lacking.

Less costly options for her remaining teeth might involve no treatment or a minimalist approach, more appropriate for end-of-life care, consisting of denture remake/reline, interim therapeutic restorations for caries, antibiotics for symptomatic endodontic infection, and chlorhexidine swabs for periodontal infections. These options were ruled out because of her high function and life expectancy of more than 12 years. Maria was happy with the aesthetics of the immediate CDs. Unfortunately, she was disappointed in the function of the mandibular CD for the first 6 months while awaiting osseointegration. After 6 months, we exposed the implants and placed overdenture abutments (see **Fig. 5**E). We retrofitted her mandibular CD to the new abutments, after which she felt an immediate improvement, and was happy with the final results (see **Fig. 5**F).

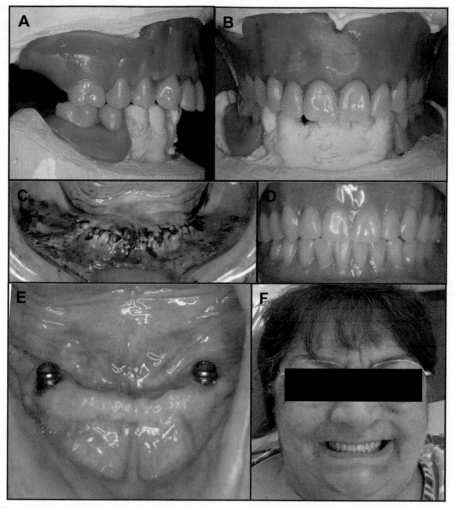

Fig. 5. Treatment photos. (*A, B*) Wax-up to dentures with appropriate vertical dimension and good support of facial muscles and lips. (*C*) After extractions and immediate implant placements, showing adequate hemostasis despite warfarin therapy. (*D*) After surgery, with immediate complete dentures (CDs) in mouth. (*E*) Six months postoperatively, overdenture abutments were placed. Mandibular CD was modified and retrofitted to abutments. (*F*) Six months postoperatively, with final modified CDs.

SUMMARY

The older patient often presents with clinically challenging dental problems and complex medical, social, psychological, and financial barriers to oral health. With careful consideration, the clinician must design a thoughtfully sequenced treatment plan that addresses the dental condition and facilitates improved oral health. This article presents several models and a summary of treatment-planning considerations that serve to guide the clinician in this endeavor.

As the case of Maria evinces, age alone does not dictate the course of dental disease. She required several alterations to her treatment stemming from a compromised medical condition, disability, and impending cognitive decline. The combination of these factors may well put her at greater risk for frailty, and thus precipitate the need for greater modifications during future treatment. Flexibility and good communication during the treatment-planning process ameliorated her aesthetic concerns and ultimately led to a successful outcome.

REFERENCES

1. Vincent GK, Velkoff VA. The next four decades, the older population in the United States: 2010 to 2050, current population reports. Washington, DC: U.S. Census Bureau; 2010. p. 1–4.
2. MacArthur Foundation Research Network on an Aging Society. Facts and fictions about an aging America. Contexts 2009;8:16–21.
3. Kinsella K, He W. U.S. Census Bureau, international population reports, P95/09-1, an aging world: 2008. Washington, DC: U.S. Government Printing Office; 2009.
4. Werner CA. The older population: 2010, 2010 census briefs. Washington, DC: U.S. Census Bureau; 2011. p. 1–19.
5. An G, Douglass CW, Monopoli M. Considerations for dental treatment in long-term care facilities. J Mass Dent Soc 2003;52:28–32.
6. Lee WC, Dooley KE, Ory MG, et al. Meeting the geriatric workforce shortage for long-term care: opinions from the field. Gerontol Geriatr Educ 2013;34:354–71.
7. Chapman DP, Williams SM, Strine TW, et al. Dementia and its implications for public health. Prev Chronic Dis 2006;3(2):A34. Available at: http://www.cdc.gov/pcd/issues/2006/apr/toc.htm. Accessed November 13, 2012.
8. Kane RL, Talley KM, Shamliyan T, et al. Common syndromes in older adults related to primary and secondary prevention. Evidence Report/Technology Assessment No. 87. AHRQ Publication No. 11-05157-EF-1. Rockville (MD): Agency for Healthcare Research and Quality; 2011.
9. National Center for Health Statistics. Health, United States, 2012: with special feature on emergency care. Hyattsville (MD): 2013.
10. Freedman V, Martin LG, Schoeni RF. Recent trends in disability and functioning among older adults in the United States, a systematic review. JAMA 2002;288:3137–46.
11. Kelly JE, Van Kirk LE, Garst CC. Decayed, missing, and filled teeth in adults. US: National Health Survey, 1960–62. National Center for Health Statistics. Vital Health Stat 1975;11(23).
12. Beltrán-Aguilar ED, Barker LK, Canto MT, et al, Centers for Disease Control and Prevention. Surveillance for dental caries, dental sealants, tooth retention, edentulism, and enamel fluorosis—United States, 1988–1994 and 1999–2002. MMWR Surveill Summ 2005;54(3):1–44.
13. Griffin SO, Jones JA, Brunson D, et al. Burden of oral disease among older adults and implications for public health priorities. Am J Public Health 2012;102:411–8.
14. Douglass CW, Shih A, Ostry L. Will there be a need for complete dentures in the United States in 2020? J Prosthet Dent 2002;87:5–8.
15. Eke PI, Dye BA, Wei L, et al. Prevalence of periodontitis in adults in the United States: 2009 and 2010. J Dent Res 2012;91:914–20.
16. Dye BA, Li X, Beltrán-Aguilar ED. Selected oral health indicators in the United States, 2005–2008. NCHS data brief, no 96. Hyattsville (MD): National Center for Health Statistics; 2012.

17. Oong EM, Griffin SO, Presson S, et al. Estimates of dry mouth in adult U.S. Population, NHANES 1999-2002. J Dent Res 2007;86A:961. Available at: www.dentalresearch.org.

18. Nasseh K, Vujicic M. Dental care utilization continues to decline among working-age adults, increases among the elderly, stable among children. Health Policy Resources Center Research Brief. Chicago (IL): American Dental Association; 2013. Available at: http://www.ada.org/sections/professionalResources/pdfs/HPRCBrief_1013_2.pdf. Accessed November 11, 2013.

19. Macek MD, Manski RJ, Vargas CM, et al. Comparing oral health care utilization estimates in the United States across three nationally representative surveys. Health Serv Res 2002;37:499–521.

20. American Dental Association, Survey Center. 2007 oral health care of vulnerable elderly, patients survey. Chicago (IL): ADA News; 2009. p. 1–25. Available at: https://www.ada.org/sections/publicResources/pdfs/oral_elderly_survey.pdf. Accessed November 13, 2013.

21. Hook R, Comer RW, Trombly RM, et al. Treatment planning process in dental schools. J Dent Educ 2002;66:68–74.

22. Glick M, Siegel MA, Brightman VJ. Evaluation of the dental patient: diagnosis and medical risk assessment. In: Greenberg MS, Glick M, editors. Burket's oral medicine diagnosis and treatment. 10th edition. Hamilton (Canada): BC Decker Inc; 2003. p. 5–33.

23. Dounis G, Ditmyer MM, McClain MA, et al. Preparing the workforce for oral disease prevention in an aging population. J Dent Educ 2010;74:1086–94.

24. Laudenbach JM. Treatment planning for the geriatric patient. In Clinician's guide to oral health in geriatric patients. 3rd edition. Edmonds (WA): American Academy of Oral Medicine; 2010. p. 7–8.

25. Ettinger RL. Rational dental care: part 1. Has the concept changed in 20 years? J Can Dent Assoc 2006;72:441–5.

26. Chen X, Clark JJ. Multidimensional risk assessment for tooth loss in a geriatric population with diverse medical and dental backgrounds. J Am Geriatr Soc 2011;59:1116–22.

27. Niessen LC, Wetle T, Wirthman GP. Clinical management of the cognitively impaired older adult. In: Holm-Pedersen P, Loe H, editors. Textbook of geriatric dentistry. 2nd edition. Copenhagen (Denmark): Munksgaard; 1996. p. 248–57.

28. Cottone JA. Treatment planning concepts. In: Bricker SL, Langlais RP, Miller CS, editors. Oral diagnosis, oral medicine, and treatment planning. 2nd edition. Philadelphia: Lea & Febiger; 1994. p. 783–4.

29. Durso SC. Interaction with other health team members in caring for elderly patients. Dent Clin North Am 2005;49:377–88.

30. Shay K. Identifying the needs of the elderly dental patient. The geriatric dental assessment. Dent Clin North Am 1994;38:499–523.

31. Ettinger RL. Meeting the oral health needs to promote the well-being of the geriatric population: educational research issues. J Dent Educ 2010;74:29–35.

32. Berkey DB, Shay K, Holm-Pedersen P. Clinical decision-making for the elderly dental patient. In: Holm-Pedersen P, Loe H, editors. Textbook of geriatric dentistry. 2nd edition. Copenhagen (Denmark): Munksgaard; 1996. p. 319–37.

33. Ettinger RL. Rational dental care: part 2. A case history. J Can Dent Assoc 2006; 72:447–52.

34. Johnson TE, Shuman SK, Ofstehage JC. Treatment planning for the geriatric dental patient. Dent Clin North Am 1997;41:945–59.

35. Mulligan R, Vanderlinde MA. Treating the older adult dental patient: what are the issues of Concern. J Calif Dent Assoc 2009;37:804–10.
36. Lo B. Assessing decision-making capacity. Law Med Health Care 1990;18(3): 193–201.
37. Karlawish JH, Pearlman RA. Determination of decision-making capacity. In: Cassel CK, Leipzig RM, Cohen HJ, et al, editors. Geriatric medicine: an evidence-based approach. 4th edition. New York: Springer-Verlag; 2003. p. 1233–41.
38. Wirshing DA, Wirshing WC, Marder SR, et al. Informed consent: assessment of comprehension. Am J Psychiatry 1998;155:1508–11.
39. Moy J, Marson DC. Assessment of decision-making capacity in older adults: an emerging area of practice and research. J Gerontol B Psychol Sci Soc Sci 2007; 62B:3–11.
40. Sfikas PM. A duty to disclose, issues to consider in securing informed consent. J Am Dent Assoc 2003;134:1329–33.
41. Zimring SD. Health care decision-making capacity: a legal perspective for long-term care providers. J Am Med Dir Assoc 2006;7:322–6.
42. Link BG, Phelan JO. Social conditions as fundamental causes of disease. J Health Soc Behav 1995;(Spec No):80–94.
43. Metcalf SS, Northridge ME, Lamster IB. A systems perspective for dental health in older adults. Am J Public Health 2011;101:1820–2.
44. Dumitrescu AL, Toma C, Lascu V. Self-liking, self-competence, body investment and perfectionism: associations with oral health status and oral-health-related behaviors. Oral Health Prev Dent 2009;7:191–200.
45. Mesas AE, de Andrade SM, Cabrera MA. Factors associated with negative self-perception of oral health among elderly people in a Brazilian community. Gerodontology 2008;25:49–56.
46. Friedlander AH, Friedlander IK, Gallas M, et al. Late-life depression: its oral health significance. Int Dent J 2003;53:41–50.
47. Bender IB, Bender AB. Diabetes mellitus and the dental pulp. J Endod 2003;29: 383–9.
48. Negrato CA, Tarzia O, Jovanovic L, et al. Periodontal disease and diabetes mellitus. J Appl Oral Sci 2013;21:1–12.
49. Huang DL, Chan KC, Young BA. Poor oral health and quality of life in older U.S. adults with diabetes mellitus. J Am Geriatr Soc 2013;31:1782–8.
50. Fouad AF, Burleson J. The effect of diabetes mellitus on endodontic treatment outcomes: data from an electronic patient record. J Am Dent Assoc 2003;134: 43–51.
51. Lockhart PB, Bolger AF, Papapanou PN, et al. Periodontal disease and athero-sclerotic vascular disease: does the evidence support an independent association? A scientific statement from the American Heart Association. Circulation 2012;125:2520–44.
52. Turner MD, Ship JA. Dry mouth and its effects on the oral health of elderly people. J Am Dent Assoc 2007;138:15s–20s.
53. Fried LP, Ferrucci L, Darer J, et al. Untangling the concepts of disability, frailty, and comorbidity: implications for improved targeting and care. J Gerontol A Biol Sci Med Sci 2004;59:255–63.
54. Malamed SF. Angina pectoris. Handbook of medical emergencies in the dental office. 2nd edition. St. Louis: Mosby; 1982. p. 327–8.
55. Niwa H, Sugimura M, Satoh Y, et al. Cardiovascular response to epinephrine-containing local anesthesia in patients with cardiovascular disease. Oral Surg Oral Med Oral Pathol Oral Radiol Endod 2001;92:610–6.

56. Andreotti F, Davies GJ, Hackett DR, et al. Major circadian fluctuations in fibrino-lytic factors and possible relevance to time of onset of myocardial infarction, sudden cardiac death and stroke. Am J Cardiol 1988;62:635–7.

57. Baddour LM, Bettmann MA, Bolger AF, et al. AHA Scientific Statement: nonvalv-ular cardiovascular device-related infections. Circulation 2003;108:2015–31.

58. American Academy of Orthopaedic Surgeons & American Dental Association. Prevention of orthopaedic implant infection in patients undergoing dental pro-cedures; evidence-based guideline and evidence report. AAOS Clinical Prac-tice Guideline Unit 2012; v0.2.2.2.2012:74–105. http://www.aaos.org/research/guidelines/PUDP/PUDP_guideline.pdf. Accessed December 31, 2013.

59. Takahashi K. Xerostomia and dysphagia. Clin Calcium 2012;22:59–65.

60. Langmore SE, Skarupski KA, Park PS, et al. Predictors of aspiration pneumonia in nursing home residents. Dysphagia 2002;17:298–307.

61. Kollef MH. Prevention of hospital-associated pneumonia and ventilator-associated pneumonia. Crit Care Med 2004;32:1396–405.

62. DeRiso AJ II, Ladowski JS, Dillon TA, et al. Chlorhexidine gluconate 0.12% oral rinse reduces the incidence of total nosocomial respiratory infection and non-prophylactic systemic antibiotic use in patients undergoing heart surgery. Chest 1996;109:1556–61.

63. Brennan MT, Hong C, Furney SL, et al. Utility of an international normalized ratio testing device in a hospital-based dental practice. J Am Dent Assoc 2008;139:697–703.

64. Jeske AH, Suchko GD. Lack of a scientific basis for routine discontinuation of oral anticoagulation therapy before dental treatment. J Am Dent Assoc 2003;134:1492–7.

65. Thomatson JM, Kelly SA, Bendkowski A, et al. Two implant retained overden-tures - a review of the literature supporting the McGill and York consensus state-ments. J Dent 2012;40:22–34.

66. The McGill consensus statement on overdentures. Quintessence Int 2003;34:78–9.

67. Hamdan NM, Gray-Donald K, Awad MA, et al. Do implant overdentures improve dietary intake? A randomized control trial. J Dent Res 2013;92:146S–53S.

68. Preciado A, Del Rio J, Suarez-Garcia MJ, et al. Differences in impact of patient and prosthetic characteristics on oral health-related quality of life among implant-retained overdenture wearers. J Dent 2012;40:857–65.

69. Muller F, Duvernay E, Loup A, et al. Implant-supported mandibular overdentures in very old adults: a randomized controlled trial. J Dent Res 2013;92:154S–60S.

Oral Health Disparity in Older Adults

Dental Decay and Tooth Loss

Paula K. Friedman, DDS, MSD, MPH[a],*, Laura B. Kaufman, DMD[a,b],
Steven L. Karpas, DMD[a]

KEYWORDS

- Dental decay • Tooth loss • Older adults • Dental care • Quality of life
- Social implications of oral health • Employment opportunities • Social inequities

KEY POINTS

- Oral health disparities exist in the aging population regarding untreated dental caries and edentulism related to income, sex, race and ethnicity, and education level.
- Access to dental care in older adults may be complicated by several factors including finances; transportation; medical and psychological complexities; and attitudes of patients, caregivers, and providers.
- Oral health has far greater implications on quality of life for older adults than generally recognized, including employment opportunities. Disparities in public policy regarding oral health for older adults nationally may compound social inequities.

INTRODUCTION

The number of older adults in the United States is increasing. The 2005 White House Conference on Aging focused on aging Baby Boomers (people born between 1946 and 1964) and their impact on the economy.[1] The conference's main agenda proposed solutions on accommodating an estimated 73 million people within this population in the next 40 years as they move into and through the older years of life. Approximately 20% of the US population will consist of those older than the age of 65 by 2040.[1]

The Surgeon General's Report on Oral Health in America created a landmark position in elevating oral health as part of overall health when it stated that oral health is a necessary component of good general health.[2] Large numbers of older adults are

[a] Department of General Dentistry, Boston University Goldman School of Dental Medicine, 72 East Concord Street, Boston, MA 02118, USA; [b] Section of Geriatrics, Boston Medical Center, Boston, MA 02118, USA
* Corresponding author. Department of General Dentistry, Boston University Goldman School of Dental Medicine, 72 East Concord Street, B330, Boston, MA 02118.
E-mail address: pkf@bu.edu

Dent Clin N Am 58 (2014) 757–770
http://dx.doi.org/10.1016/j.cden.2014.06.004
0011-8532/14/$ – see front matter © 2014 Elsevier Inc. All rights reserved.

retaining their natural teeth as they age and continue to use dental services throughout their retirement years. This trend is significant because the mouth reflects a person's health and well-being throughout life.

The benefits of retaining natural dentition include the ability to eat a healthy and varied diet and to maintain social interactions. However, the retention of natural teeth into older age puts greater numbers of teeth at risk for tooth decay and periodontal disease, because age-related issues may hamper oral hygiene efforts and the ability to access regular dental care.

The older adult population in the United States is heterogeneous, and disparities in oral health exist among those aged 65 and older. There are disparities in the rates of dental decay and tooth loss related to income, sex, race and ethnicity, and education level.[1,2]

EPIDEMIOLOGY OF EDENTULISM AND DENTAL DECAY IN OLDER ADULTS

A major source of national oral health data in the United States is the National Health and Nutrition Examination Survey (NHANES). The NHANES is an on-going series of studies conducted by the National Center for Health Statistics, a division of the US Department of Health and Human Services, Public Health Service at the Centers for Disease Control and Prevention. NHANES surveys are designed to longitudinally assess the health and nutritional status of adults and children in the United States.[2]

Before the 1999 survey, NHANES surveys were conducted periodically (ie, 1971–1974 and 1988–1994). Since 1999 the surveys are continuous and conducted annually, and up-dates are issued in 2- or 4-year cycles (1999–2004; 2005–2008). The data collected are stratified by age, race and ethnicity, poverty level, and sex. Data collected on older adults are divided into age subcategories of 65 to 74 years, and 75+ years.

The oral health portion of the surveys consists of participant interviews and clinical dental examinations. Assessments include the prevalence of dental diseases and conditions, along with demographic and socioeconomic data. Mean number of permanent teeth, caries rates, and edentulous rates have been historically assessed.

The prevalence of edentulism in older adults has been declining over the past decades from a reported 45.6% from 1971–1974 to 23% reported during the period 2005 to 2008 (**Fig. 1**).[3] This continues the trend of overall edentulous rate reduction in comparison with previously reported rates of 34% in 1988 to 1994 and 27% in 1999 to 2004.[3] The implication for dentists of declining rates of edentulism is that there will be more potential older adults retaining some or all of their natural dentition requiring dental treatment (ie, increasing need and demand for dental services by older adults in the future) (see **Fig. 1**).

Disparities in edentulous rates in older adults are related to income, age, sex, and race and ethnicity.[3] The 2005 to 2008 NHANES data reported significantly more edentulous non-Hispanic older black adults (32%) compared with Mexican-American older adults (16%) and non-Hispanic white older adults (22%).

There are significant disparities in the prevalence of edentulism inversely proportional to income level, with prevalence more than double for older adults living below 100% of the federal poverty level (37%) compared with those persons living at 200% of the poverty level or higher (16%). The lower the income level, the higher the probability of edentulism (**Fig. 2**).

PREVALENCE OF UNTREATED DENTAL CARIES IN OLDER ADULTS

Fig. 3 and **Table 1**[3–5] show prevalence of untreated caries in older adults. NHANES 2005 to 2008 reported similar results to those of NHANES 1999 to 2002. However,

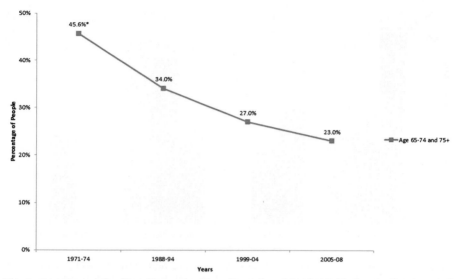

Fig. 1. Prevalence of edentulism over time. (*From* Dye BA, Li X, Beltrán-Aguilar ED, et al. Selected oral health indicators in the United States, 2005–2008. NCHS data brief, no 96. Hyattsville (MD): National Center for Health Statistics; 2012.)

there is a significant decrease in untreated caries in comparison with NHANES 1988 to 1994.[4] The prevalence of untreated caries was more than twice as high for both non-Hispanic black persons (35.8%) and Mexican-American persons (36.4%) compared with non-Hispanic whites (17.8%). There were significant differences in the prevalence of untreated dental caries in older adults living in poverty. The prevalence ranged from 41.3% for persons living below 100% of the federal poverty level to 15.3% for persons living at 200% or higher of the poverty level (see **Fig. 3**). The prevalence of overall untreated dental caries was significantly lower (15.6%) for females compared with males (25.1%).[6]

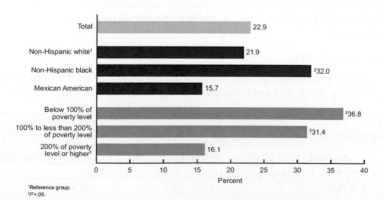

Fig. 2. Prevalence of complete tooth loss (edentulism), by race and ethnicity and poverty level among adults aged 65 and older: United States, 2005–2008. (*From* Dye BA, Li X, Beltrán-Aguilar ED, et al. Selected oral health indicators in the United States, 2005–2008. NCHS data brief, no 96. Hyattsville (MD): National Center for Health Statistics; 2012.)

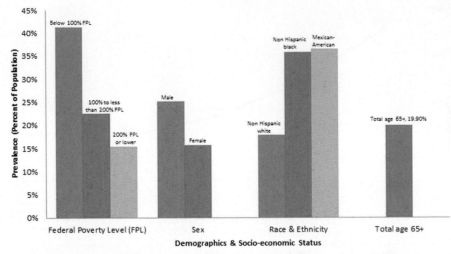

Fig. 3. Prevalence of untreated dental caries by sex, race and ethnicity, and poverty level: United States 2005–2008. (*Data from* CDC/NCHS. National Health and Nutrition Examination Survey, Table 76. Untreated dental caries, by selected characteristics: United States, selected years 1971–1974 through 2005–2008. Available at: http://www.cdc.gov/nchs/data/hus/2011/076.pdf. Accessed July 17, 2014; and Dye BA, Tan S, Thornton-Evans G, et al. Trends in oral health status: United States, 1988–1994 and 1999–2004. National Center for Health Statistics. Vital Health Stat 11 2007;(248):1–92.)

FUTURE TRENDS

The trend in older adults is for higher numbers of remaining teeth along with untreated dental caries. The challenge for the dental profession is to clarify barriers to needed treatment of older adults and work toward more accessible dental treatment for all.

ACCESS TO DENTAL CARE FOR RESIDENTS IN LONG-TERM CARE FACILITIES

The issue of inadequate oral health care for a significant segment of the US population has been framed as a problem of access. Those living in remote areas, the economically disadvantaged, those with severe medical comorbidities or other special needs, and those who are institutionalized, especially the frail elderly, have difficulty accessing dental care.[7]

Long-Term Care Facilities

As the over-65 population grows, there is a concurrent growth in the number of frail older adults living in long-term care (LTC). In 2009, 1.5 million (4.1%) of the

Table 1
National Health and Nutrition Examination Survey (NHANES)

	NHANES (2005–2008), %	NHANES (1999–2002), %	NHANES (1988–1994), %
Age 65+	19.9	—	—
Age 65–74	19.6	17	25.4
Age 75+	20.2	20.3	30.3

Data from CDC/NCHS. National Health and Nutrition Examination Survey, Table 76. Untreated dental caries, by selected characteristics: United States, selected years 1988–1994 through 2005–2008. Available at: http://www.cdc.gov/nchs/data/hus/2011/076.pdf. Accessed July 17, 2014.

65+ population lived in LTC or assisted-living facilities.[8] Oral health has been poor among older adults living in LTC, many of whom need assistance in traveling to an outside dental office or need dental care brought to them.[9] Problems caused by age-associated physiologic changes, underlying chronic diseases, and/or cognitive decline make it difficult for LTC residents to travel to outside community dental providers.[10,11]

Older adult residents of LTC pose a challenge for dentists and the dental health team. Historically, the burden of providing dental care for the aging population has fallen to private community-based dental practices and/or to those few dentists who provide onsite institutional care.[12]

Unfortunately, there are limited numbers of dentists who are willing and able to provide dental care to LTC residents.[11] Dentists may be reluctant to treat elderly patients in LTC, citing pressures from private practice, including concerns about taking time from their practices to travel to LTC. Other reasons for dentists' reluctance to treat LTC residents include the challenge of managing frail older adults with complicated physical and cognitive conditions, and the complexity of the work environment within LTC.[11,12] Furthermore, many dentists perceive themselves as inadequately trained to treat LTC residents, also citing poor remuneration from private and public dental insurances plans and/or personal negative feelings in treating people with complex medical and psychosocial conditions.

Other barriers include inadequately trained LTC staff. Historically, nurses and certified nursing assistants in LTC facilities have not been trained to provide routine oral hygiene care or to recognize dental problems. Performing oral hygiene for older adults may be considered an unpleasant task and therefore may be avoided.

All these factors put older adults at increased risk for oral diseases. As oral disease persists, it often increases in severity. Untreated dental disease can lead to acute episodes of pain, swelling, and/or bleeding, and possible tooth loss. Consequences of untreated oral disease and tooth loss include decreased chewing ability, decreased nutritional intake, altered cognitive capability, problems with speaking, diminished quality of life, possible avoidance of social interactions, and further complications of other existing chronic health issues.

Because medical and functional problems can put older adults at increased risk for oral diseases, it is crucial that these older adults receive regular professional care to reduce the impact of dental diseases on the quality of life and general health.[11]

Dentists who provide onsite clinical dental services within LTC facilities experience unique environmental nuances that compound difficult treatment decisions: complicated social surroundings, complex clinical situations, and challenging ethical issues of caring for patients with chronic disabilities.[13] Often, ideal dentistry cannot be performed because of such issues as the chronic consumption of highly refined carbohydrate liquids and foods causing ongoing recurrent decay; residents' cognitive limitations causing difficulty with patient compliance; behavior management issues; and the physical limitations involved with performing daily oral hygiene because of chronic conditions, such as arthritis or neuromuscular degenerative disorders (SLK professional observations).

INADEQUATE SUPPLY AND GEOGRAPHIC MALDISTRIBUTION OF DENTAL PROVIDERS
Inadequate Supply of Dentists

In states that include adult dental coverage in Medicaid programs, access to dental providers can still be challenging for older adults, because limited reimbursement rates serve as the primary disincentive to dentists to participate as providers.[11,12,14]

The nation currently faces a severe shortage of dental providers for underserved people.[13] Only about 20% of the nation's 179,000 practicing dentists accept Medicaid payment for dental services. Of those dentists who treat Medicaid patients, fewer than 8500 devote a substantial part of their practice to serving the poor, the chronically ill, and rural residents, many of whom reside in LTC facilities.[11,13]

The current dental workforce is challenged to meet the needs of older adults, with the US Department of Health and Human Services reporting an upcoming shortage of dentists.[10] A rapidly aging generation of dentists is not being replaced quickly enough with new graduates to avoid sharp declines in the nation's oral health workforce. The number of dental health professional shortage areas has nearly tripled from 800 in 1993 to more than 2300 in 2010. More than 49 million people live in areas categorized as Dental Health Provider Shortage Areas.[13] As the workforce shortage continues, there will be increased difficulty identifying dentists within these shortage areas willing and able to treat frail, LTC residents dependent on Medicaid programs.[13,15,16]

Maldistribution of Dentists

In addition to a looming national dentist shortage, there are fewer dentists practicing in rural communities compared with the suburbs or urban centers. The trend for graduating dentists is to locate their practices near large urban areas with dense populations to successfully build their new practices. To reverse this national trend, the federal government has encouraged dentists to locate in traditionally underserved areas via the National Health Service Corps, offering dental scholarships and/or dental school loan forgiveness programs for participants who agree to practice in Dental Health Provider Shortage Areas for a specified time. In addition, the current distribution of dentists does not adequately address access to oral health needs in an increasingly diverse population across the aging continuum. Several studies indicate that an increasingly diverse oral health workforce may be better suited to meeting the needs and demands of the increasingly diverse population.[17–19] Studies of practice profiles reflect that dentists who are from underrepresented communities tend to treat higher percentages of underrepresented, disadvantaged, lower socioeconomic patients compared with nonunderrepresented minority professional colleagues.[20,21] Patients may feel more comfortable with a provider from similar racial, ethnic, cultural, and/ or linguistic backgrounds and may therefore engage in more oral health-seeking behaviors and help reduce the oral health disparities that exist.

ECONOMICS OF DENTAL CARE

One of the greatest barriers to access to dental care for older adults is poverty.[11,12] Among older adults, poverty occurs more frequently in combination with other barriers to access to care, such as institutionalization, frailty, race, ethnicity, language/cultural issues, lack of education, lack of perceived dental need, the existence of severe medical comorbidities, and/or functional limitations.[12]

Although children's dental coverage was addressed in the Patient Protection and Affordable Care Act, older adult dental coverage was omitted.[15] Older adults usually do not have private dental insurance. Because of very high costs, only 2% of Americans maintain a dental insurance plan into the retirement years.[12,14] Lacking dental health insurance, accessing dental care becomes an out-of-pocket expense. Lack of available funds for preventive and basic dental care may lead to a significant public health issue as more people live into their later years.

Government health insurance offers few dental options for older American adults. Many veterans do not qualify for dental benefits through the Veteran's Administration.

Medicare has no provisions for preventive dental care or for routine dental procedures, providing only limited treatment deemed "medically necessary." For example, Medicare covers dental services only considered to be an integral part of a medical procedure, such as jaw reconstruction following accidental injury, or for extractions done in preparation for radiation treatment of neoplastic jaw diseases. Medicare sometimes pays for a dental examination, but not treatment, preceding kidney or heart valve transplantation.[15,16,22]

OBSTACLES TO OLDER ADULT DENTAL CARE

As the older adult population continues to grow, the demand for LTC will continue to rise (**Table 2**).[10,23,24] Many within this population have maintained their dentition into older age, and will expect continued oral care as they age.[25] One proposal to provide oral care for LTC residents is to use alternate providers to deliver care at a lower cost than dentists. A new midlevel dental provider, the dental health aide therapist (also known as a dental therapist), has been recently introduced in limited geographic US regions (Alaska, Minnesota) as an experiment in increasing access to care for underserved populations. In the United States, dental therapists are trained and licensed to deliver limited diagnostic, preventive, and restorative oral health care in collaboration with licensed dentists.[25] Additional innovative models may include having members of the medical health care team as providers of some preventive and primary care treatment services (eg, fluoride varnish application, oral cancer screening, preliminary oral examination) to strengthen the oral health–systemic health link and concurrently increase access to care.

SOCIAL IMPLICATIONS OF TOOTH LOSS AND TOOTH DECAY IN THE ELDERLY
Impact on Employment

The World Health Organization Active Aging approach encourages strategies to keep older people socially engaged and productive.[26] Providing preventive, diagnostic,

Table 2	
Obstacles to older adult dental care	
Patients' Perspective	**Dentist Perspective**
• Lack of perceived need for care	• Age biases
• Limited finances	• Low remuneration from Medicaid
• Cultural preferences/language barriers	• Cumbersome Medicaid administrative
• Accessibility of dental care	paperwork
• Transportation issues to dental office	• Medicaid preauthorization in some
• Availability of dental care	treatments
• Cognitive impairments	• Excessive time to treat relative to low fees
• Mobility issues	• Lack training to treat frail elderly
• Caretaker stress	• Too disruptive to schedule
• Social isolation	• Dislike by dentist, staff and other patients
• Fear	• Patients are too emotionally labile
• Distrust/Dislike of dentists	• High no-show/cancellation rate
• Low socioeconomic status	• Lack of handicap access to office
• Limited education of LTC staff, nurses, families and patients on need for oral healthcare	• Office physical barriers limiting safe patient wheel-chair transfer into dental chair
	• Limited evidence-based dental care guidelines
	• Limited number of dentists trained in geriatric dentistry

Data from Refs.[10,23,24]

primary, and advanced dental services to aging adults has significant societal implications. There is an increasing urgency in the demographic imperative to find ways to keep older adults functioning independently in the community and adding quality to their lives.

Older adults stay involved in the workplace, politically and socially. The average age of workers is increasing.[27] Studies have shown that continued employment provides a sense of self-worth and social engagement, both of which are predictors of successful aging. Conversely, loss of employment can lead to social isolation, depression, and even thoughts of suicide. Many men and women continue to work beyond the usual retirement age of 65 (or sometimes earlier, depending on contractual arrangements) (**Fig. 4**).

The US Census Bureau Population Bulletin, based on data from the Bureau of Labor Statistics, shows that since about 1985, both men and women older than age 65 have increased participation in the US labor force each year.[28] Men between the ages of 65 and 69 are approaching 40% participation, and women between ages 65 and 69 are approaching 30% participation. Therefore, even if someone of retirement age is financially comfortable, there may be strong social drivers keeping him or her in the work environment. Appearance is important in the workplace, including the appearance of one's smile. Older adults will be increasingly interested in replacing missing teeth with implants, accessing esthetic dentistry, and restoring decayed and broken teeth to maintain oral health and youthful appearance.[29]

Not everyone can afford to retire, even if that were their desire. Many older adults fear outliving their savings, pensions, or social security benefits, so the incentive to

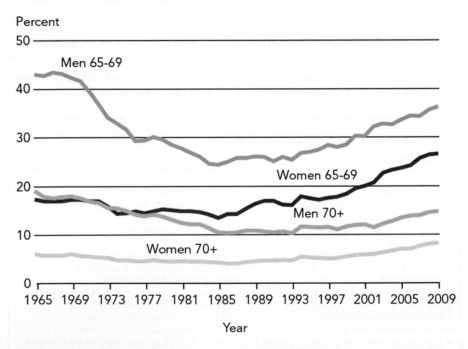

Note: Estimates are based on a survey of the population and are subject to both sampling and nonsampling error.

Fig. 4. Labor force participation rates of men and women ages 65 and older, 1965 to 2009. (*From* Bureau of Labor Statistics, Current Population Surveys. Available at: http://www.bls.gov/cps/. Accessed December 12, 2013.)

supplement those financial resources with income from work (full-time or part-time) is keeping people in the workforce well past the traditional retirement age. Maintenance of a healthy dentition is important to gainful employment, especially in jobs that require interacting with the public. In the economy since 2008, older adults have faced difficult challenges in finding employment.[30–33] An October 2009 *New York Times* article stated, "In fact, there are more Americans 65 and older in the job market today than at any time in history, 6.6 million, compared with 4.1 million in 2001."[34] For older adults who seek employment, having missing, broken, or decayed teeth may be a deterrent to being hired, and may detract from the interview process. The importance of the appearance of teeth in relation to employment was reinforced when, after a multiyear moratorium on restorative services for adults under Medicaid in Massachusetts, coverage for anterior composites was recently reinstated, presumably because of the impact that healthy dentition has on employability for adults.

Quality of Life

When asked to identify the functions of teeth, professionals and the lay public easily can name the "big three"[35,36]: (1) eating and mastication, (2) appearance and self-esteem, and (3) speech and phonation. There are several other, equally important functions of the dentition that contribute to quality of life that may not come to mind as quickly. All of the following were volunteered responses from older adult audiences attending oral health presentations when asked, "Why are teeth important?":

- Playing brass or woodwind musical instruments
- Playing a harmonica
- Singing
- Whistling
- Kissing
- Self-defense (biting)
- Opening beer bottles (input from a patient) (**Fig. 5**)

Good oral health may be a significant predictor of quality of life in older adults. The social implications of the previously mentioned activities and how they relate to keeping older adults (or individuals of any age) actively involved and engaged in a community are evident. The joy of singing with a community or spiritual choir; of playing a trumpet, clarinet, oboe, saxophone, trombone with a local orchestra or jazz band; of whistling as one walks down the street on a crisp autumn day; of embracing a loved one and touching your lips to theirs—all are more difficult if not impossible without teeth. Patients have described how they have fended off attackers by biting them (a function of teeth that had not typically been listed among the "big three" in dental school!).

The literature describes how missing teeth or teeth in poor repair can lead to embarrassment, withdrawal, and social isolation.[37–40] However, adults do not need a full complement of teeth to function. In a seminal study, Elias and Sheiham discuss that many people may be satisfied with less than 28 natural teeth in the analysis of the shortened dental arch concept.[41] Thus partial edentulism in the older adult, especially in the posterior segment of the arch, may not impact quality of life **Box 1**.

SOCIAL IMPLICATIONS OF DISPARITIES IN ACCESS OR ORAL HEALTH CARE FOR OLDER ADULTS

Access to oral health services may be a function of education, income, location, transportation, culture, beliefs, and third-party coverage.[42,43] Medicare, a health insurance

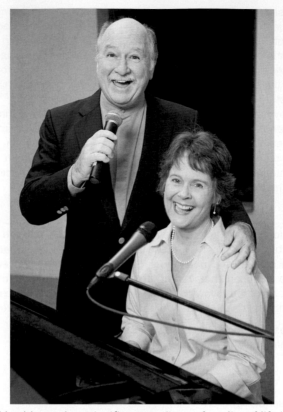

Fig. 5. Good oral health may be a significant predictor of quality of life in older adults.

program provided for citizens 65 and older and federally funded, provides no dental coverage. Medicaid, a health insurance program for low income–eligible individuals and families, requires that dental services be provided to children to the age of 21. After the age of 21, it is at the discretion of states to determine what, if any, dental services are provided to adults.[44] In 2011, seven states reported no adult dental benefits under Medicaid, 19 states reported comprehensive dental benefits for adults under Medicaid, and the remaining states provided varying levels of coverage for adults.[44] The cost of health care services provided under Medicaid is shared between the State and the Federal Governments.

Clearly, those low-income residents of states with comprehensive dental services under Medicaid have potentially greater access to care than low-income residents in states with no adult dental services. But health promotion is multifactorial, including fluoridation of pubic water supplies, distribution of dentists, and a state oral health plan that includes adults. Individual belief systems contribute powerfully to how the constellation of variables, including diet and personal oral hygiene practices, result in the oral status of any person.

The presence or absence of teeth is not just related to esthetics and function. Bergdahl and colleagues[43] conducted a study on the relationship between the presence or absence of teeth in humans and cognitive functioning and found that, even after controlling for important associated factors, such as age, gender, education level, living conditions, occupation, stress, diseases, and socioeconomic status, the

> **Box 1**
> **Case report**
>
> Mary McCrory was referred for a dental consultation and evaluation for denture fabrication. Mary is an 80-year-old Irish immigrant who has lived in Boston for the past 60 years. Before moving to Boston, she lived in London in Buckingham Palace with her mother where they both worked as scullery maids in the kitchen. Mary's past medical history (PMH) is significant only for the diagnosis of agoraphobia. She has not been out of her home for the past 3 years. All meals are delivered to her. She has a homemaker twice a week, and a home health aide five times a week to provide personal care services. Her intraoral examination reveals edentulous maxillary and mandibular arches. Mary reports that she lost her dentures about 3.5 years ago when they were mistakenly thrown away during a brief hospitalization. Mary seems oriented as to place and time, knows appropriate responses to questions regarding topical issues, and in general seems pleasant and cooperative. When we discussed the possibility of fabricating a new set of dentures, she seemed interested but indicated that she was reluctant to come to our office for the visits. We told her that we were able to conduct the visits in her home.
>
> After fabricating the dentures and delivering them to Mary, she was very satisfied and gave us a broad smile. When we returned for a postinsertion visit, Mary told us that she was volunteering at a local senior center as an arts and crafts assistant.
>
> We will never know whether there was a direct correlation between the denture fabrication and Mary's volunteerism, but the literature suggests that there may have been some relationship between the absence of teeth and a sense of self-consciousness on the part of the patient.
>
> This is an actual case, although the name has been changed to protect the patient's identity.

presence of natural teeth in humans is related to higher cognitive functioning. They infer that natural teeth and mastication can be important for cognitive function, but the mechanisms remain unclear.

SUMMARY

Progress has been made in reducing dental caries and edentulism in older adults, but disparities continue to exist related to race, ethnicity, socioeconomic level, and sex. Lack of training in treating medically complex patients, economic factors including absence of coverage for oral health services in Medicare and as a required service for adults in Medicaid, and attitudinal issues on the part of patients, caregivers, and providers contribute to barriers to care for older adults. In addition to the impact of oral health on overall health, oral health impacts quality of life and social and employment opportunities.

REFERENCES

1. US Department of Health and Human Services. Oral health in America: a report of the surgeon general. Rockville (MD): US Department of Health and Human Services, National Institute of Dental and Craniofacial Research, National Institutes of Health; 2000. Available at: http://www.surgeongeneral.gov/library/reports/oralhealth/.
2. Massachusetts Department of Public Health, Office of Oral Health. The status of oral disease in Massachusetts: a great unmet need 2009. Boston: Department of Public Health; 2009. Available at: http://www.mass.gov/eohhs/docs/dph/com-health/oral-health-burden.pdf.

3. Dye BA, Li X, Beltrán-Aguilar ED, et al. Selected oral health indicators in the United States, 2005–2008. NCHS data brief, no 96. Hyattsville (MD): National Center for Health Statistics; 2012.

4. CDC/NCHS. National Health and Nutrition Examination Survey, Table 76. Untreated dental caries, by selected characteristics: United States, selected years 1971-1974 through 2005-2008. Available at: http://www.cdc.gov/nchs/data/hus/2011/076.pdf. Accessed July 17, 2014.

5. Dye BA, Tan S, Thornton-Evans G, et al. Trends in oral health status: United States, 1988-1994 and 1999-2004. National Center for Health Statistics. Vital Health Stat 11 2007;(248):1–92.

6. Dye B, Barker L, Li X, et al. Overview and quality assurance for the oral health component of the National Health and Nutrition Examination Survey (NHANES), 2005-2008. J Public Health Dent 2011;71:54–61 American Association of Public Health Dentistry.

7. Dolan TA, Atchison K, Huynh TN. Access to dental care among older adults in the United States. J Dent Educ 2005;69(9):961–74.

8. A profile of older Americans: 2011 Administration on Aging US Department of Health + Human Services. Available at: www.aoa.gov/Aging_Statistics/Profile/index.aspx. Accessed July 17, 2014.

9. US Department of Health and Human Services. Oral health in America: a report of the surgeon general. Rockville (MD): U.S. Department of Health and Human Services, National Institute of Dental and Craniofacial Research, National Institutes of Health; 2000. Available at: http://silk.nih.gov/public/hck1ocv.@www.surgeon.fullrpt.pdf.

10. Kiyak H, Reichmuth M. Barriers to and enablers of older adults' use of dental services. J Dent Educ 2005;69(9):975–86.

11. Health Professional Shortage Areas (HPSAs). 2013. Available at: http://bhpr.hrsa.gov/shortage/hpsas/. Accessed July 17, 2014.

12. MacEntee MI, Pruksapong M, Wyatt C. Insights from students following an educational rotation through dental geriatrics. J Dent Educ 2005;69(12):1368–75.

13. Guay AH. Access to dental care: the triad of essential factors in access-to-care programs. J Am Dent Assoc 2004;135:779–85.

14. A state of decay: Oral Health America. 2013. Available at: http://www.oralhealthamerica.org/pdf/StateofDecayFinal.pdf. Accessed July 17, 2014.

15. State Oral Health Workforce. 2010. Available at: http://bhpr.hrsa.gov/grants/dentistry/abstracts/2010oralhealth.html. Accessed July 17, 2014.

16. Oral Health Workforce. 2010. Available at: http://www.hrsa.gov/publichealth/clinical/oralhealth/workforce.html. Accessed July 17, 2014.

17. Evans CA, Kleinman DV, Maas WR, et al. Oral health in America: a report of the Surgeon General. Rockville (MD): US Dept of Health and Human Services, National Institutes of Health, National Institute of Dental and Craniofacial Research; 2000.

18. Sullivan LW. Missing persons: minorities in the health professions. Washington, DC: Sullivan Commission; 2004.

19. Institute of Medicine Committee on Understanding and Eliminating Racial and Ethnic Disparities in Health Care. Unequal treatment: confronting racial and ethnic disparities in health care. Washington, DC: National Academy Press; 2002.

20. Solomon ES, Williams CR, Sinkford JC. Practice location characteristics of black dentists in Texas. J Dent Educ 2001;65:571–4.

21. Brown LJ, Wagner KS, Johns B. Racial/ethnic variations of practicing dentists. JADA 2000;131:1750–4.

22. Medicare Dental Coverage page last modified July 15, 2013. Available at: http://www.cms.gov/Medicare/Coverage/MedicareDentalCoverage/index.html?redirect=/MedicareDentalCoverage. Accessed July 17, 2014.
23. Yellowitz JA. Access, place of residence and interdisciplinary opportunities. In: Lamster IB, Northridge ME, editors. Improving oral health for the elderly: an interdisciplinary approach. New York: Springer Publishing Co; 2008. p. 55–7.
24. Smith B, Ghezzi E, Manz M, et al. Oral healthcare access and adequacy in alternative long-term care facilities. Spec Care Dentist 2010;30(3):85–94.
25. Nash DA, Friedman JW, Kardos TB. Dental therapist: a global perspective. Int Dent J 2008;58(2):61–70.
26. Papadaki E, Anastassiadou V. Elderly complete denture wearers: a social approach to tooth loss. Gerodontology 2012;29:e721–7.
27. Maurer TJ. Career-relevant learning and development, worker age, and beliefs about self-efficacy for development. J Manag 2001;27:123–40.
28. Jacobsen LA, Kent M, Lee M, et al. America's aging population. Popul Bull 2011;66(1):1–18.
29. Chalmers JM, Ettinger RL. Public health issues in geriatric dentistry in the United States. Dent Clin North Am 2008;52:423–46.
30. Sedensky M. For jobless over 50, a challenging search for work. Chicago, IL: Associated Press; 2013. Available at: http://www.apnorc.org/news-media/Pages/News+Media/for-jobless-over-a-challenging-search-for-work.aspx.
31. Yarrow A. Unemployed and retired. You, too, can double dip. The Fiscal Times 2011. Available at: http://www.thefiscaltimes.com/Articles/2011/08/17/Unemployed-and-Retired-You-too-Can-Double-Dip.
32. Ansberry C. Elderly emerge as a new class of workers – and the jobless. The Wall Street Journal 2009. Available at: http://online.wsj.com/news/articles/SB123535088586444925.
33. Tugend A. Unemployed and older, and facing a jobless future. The New York Times 2013. Available at: http://www.nytimes.com/2013/07/27/your-money/unemployed-and-older-and-facing-a-jobless-future.html.
34. Greenhouse S. 65 and up and looking for work. The New York Times 2009. Available at: http://www.nytimes.com/2009/10/24/business/economy/24older.html?_r=0#.
35. Mesas AE, Andrade SM, Cabrera MA. Factors associated with negative self-perception of oral health among elderly people in a Brazilian community. Gerodontology 2008;25:49–56.
36. Locker D. Self-esteem and socioeconomic disparities in self-perceived oral health. J Public Health Dent 2009;69:1–8.
37. Thorstensson H, Johansson B. Does oral health say anything about survival in later life? Findings in a Swedish cohort of 80+ years at baseline. Community Dent Oral Epidemiol 2009;37:325–32.
38. Cousson PY, Bessadet M, Nicolas E, et al. Nutritional status, dietary intake and oral quality of life in elderly complete denture wearers. Gerodontology 2012;29:e685–92.
39. Rodrigues SM, Oliveira AC, Vargas AM, et al. Implications of edentulism on quality of life among elderly. Int J Environ Res Public Health 2012;9:100–9.
40. Warren JJ, Watkins CA, Cowen HJ, et al. Tooth loss in the very old: 13-15-year incidence among elderly Iowans. Community Dent Oral Epidemiol 2002;30:29–37.
41. Elias AC, Sheiham A. The relationship between satisfaction with mouth and number and position of teeth. J Oral Rehabil 1998;25:649–61.
42. Teofilo LT, Leles CR. Patients' self-perceived impacts and prosthodontic needs at the time and after tooth loss. Braz Dent J 2007;18(2):91–6.

43. Bergdahl M, Habib R, Bergdahl J, et al. Natural teeth and cognitive function in humans. Scand J Psychol 2007;48:557–65.
44. Oral Health America. State of decay: are older Americans coming of age without oral healthcare? 2013. Available at: http://s.bsd.net/teeth/default/page/-/SOD Update10.15.pdf. Accessed July 17, 2014.

Oral Health Disparities in Older Adults

Oral Bacteria, Inflammation, and Aspiration Pneumonia

Frank A. Scannapieco, DMD, PhD[a],*, Kenneth Shay, DDS, MS[b]

KEYWORDS

- Oral hygiene • Oral bacteria • Aspiration pneumonia • Elderly
- Vulnerable population

KEY POINTS

- The oral microflora—and the role of oral care in limiting it—has become recently appreciated; the bacteria that often contribute to initiation of pneumonia have been shown to colonize the oral cavity.
- Methods to improve oral hygiene, particularly rinses such as chlorhexidine, can reduce the risk for pneumonia in vulnerable populations.
- There is a need to educate both patients and care providers about the importance of oral hygiene to prevent pneumonia.

INTRODUCTION

Pneumonia is an inflammatory condition of the lung parenchyma, usually initiated by the introduction of bacteria or viruses into the lower airway. The initiation of pneumonia depends on the aspiration of infectious agents from proximal sites, including the oral and nasal cavities.[1] This disease is particularly prevalent in the elderly, especially those in institutions such as nursing homes, and those with several important risk factors. The role of the oral microflora in this process—and the role of oral care in limiting it—has become much more appreciated over the past decade; the bacteria that often contribute to disease initiation have been shown to colonize the oral cavity.

Pneumonia can be classified according to the location of the origin of the etiologic infectious agents (ie, from the community vs from within the institution—so-called nosocomial pneumonia). One specific form of pneumonia, aspiration pneumonia

[a] Department of Oral Biology, School of Dental Medicine, University at Buffalo - The State University of New York, Foster Hall, Buffalo, NY 14214, USA; [b] Geriatrics and Extended Care Services (10P4G), US Department of Veterans Affairs, PO Box 134002, Ann Arbor, MI 48113-4002, USA
* Corresponding author.
E-mail address: fas1@buffalo.edu

Dent Clin N Am 58 (2014) 771–782
http://dx.doi.org/10.1016/j.cden.2014.06.005   dental.theclinics.com

(AP), is an infectious process caused by the aspiration of oropharyngeal secretions colonized by pathogenic bacteria.[2] This is differentiated from aspiration pneumonitis, which is typically caused by chemical injury after inhalation of sterile gastric contents. AP can also be community acquired or acquired from the health care delivery environment, and it is common in the nursing home setting. AP is almost always caused by a mixed infection, including anaerobic bacteria derived from the oral cavity (gingival crevice), and often develops in patients with elevated risk of aspiration of oral contents into the lung, such as those with dysphagia or depressed consciousness.[1,3]

This article reviews aspects of the epidemiology, pathogenesis, and prevention of AP. In particular, the role of oral health status in the pathogenesis and prevention of the disease is highlighted.

EPIDEMIOLOGY

Pneumonia is a common disease. Together with influenza, pneumonia was the eighth most common cause of death in the United States in 2011.[4] Classification of pneumonia is based on the residence of the victim at the time of the initiation of the infection. Thus, community-acquired pneumonias are those where the infection is contracted within the community. A recent report found the crude and age-adjusted incidences of pneumonia were 6.71 and 9.43 cases per 1000 person-years (10-year risk was 6.15%).[5] The 30-day and 1-year mortality were found to be 16.5% and 31.5%, respectively. Interestingly, 62% of pneumonia cases occurred in adults older than 65. It is clear that pneumonia is a common disease with severe consequences, especially for the elderly.

Pneumonia occurring in an individual longer than 48 hours after admission to a hospital or other residential health care facility (such as a nursing home) is defined as nosocomial pneumonia.

Pneumonia is the second most common nosocomial infection in the United States (after urinary tract infection), representing 10% to 15% of these infections and is associated with substantial morbidity and mortality,[6] and cost.[7] Most patients who contract nosocomial pneumonia are infants, young children, and persons older than 65; persons who have severe underlying disease, immunosuppression, neurologic deficit, and/or cardiovascular disease; and patients undergoing abdominal surgery.

Over the past decade, as the delivery of medical care has shifted from the hospital to outpatient facilities (for delivery of services such as antibiotic therapy, cancer chemotherapy, wound management, outpatient dialysis centers, etc), the classification scheme for pneumonia has changed. Pneumonia often occurs within such health care delivery settings, but may not be so recognized. For this reason, a new term, health care–associated pneumonia,[8] has entered the literature to describe the range of patients that could be affected.

An important type of health care–associated pneumonia is nursing home–associated pneumonia (NHAP), the most common infection affecting nursing home residents.[9] NHAP is the leading cause of death in the nursing home population.[10] Its incidence among long-term care residents has been variously estimated as 0.7 to 1 episodes per 1000 patient days.[11] Mortality has been estimated to be 8% to 54%.[11] Pneumonia is the most common reason for transfer of nursing home residents to the hospital.[10] However, hospital-based treatment of NHAP is costly, which has driven practitioners to provide treatment in the nursing home rather than after transfer of the patient to the hospital. There is evidence to show that there are no differences in outcomes when comparing NHAP treated by use of oral antibiotics in the nursing home versus parenteral treatment after hospitalization.[12]

Another factor discouraging transfer to the hospital of nursing home residents with pneumonia is that the hospital environment also predisposes to pulmonary infection. Hospital-acquired pneumonia is a common infection in the hospital, often causing considerable morbidity and mortality, as well as extending the hospital stay and increasing the cost of hospital care. Pneumonia is the most common infection in the intensive care unit (ICU) setting, accounting for 10% of infections in the ICU.[13] Hospital-acquired pneumonia can be further divided into 2 subtypes: Ventilator-associated pneumonia (VAP) and non-VAP.

RISK FACTORS

Dysphagia (swallowing dysfunction) is among the most important risk factors for AP. Dysphagia is a relatively common finding in elderly, especially those in nursing homes,[14] where it can be a result of Parkinson disease, Alzheimer disease, stroke, other neurodegenerative conditions, or advanced aging.[15] A recent systematic review that sought to identify risk factors for AP found dysphagia to have a robust positive correlation with AP (odds ratio [OR], 9.84; 95% CI, 4.15–23.33).[16] In a prospective study of 189 elderly veterans residing in a Department of Veterans Affairs nursing home, significant predictors for AP included dependence for feeding, dependence for oral care, tube feeding, current smoking, multiple medical diagnoses, number of medications, and number of decayed teeth.[17] Another study that followed 358 institutionalized veterans aged 55 years and older found significant risk factors for AP for patients with no natural teeth included chronic obstructive pulmonary disease, diabetes, dependence with feeding, and presence of *Staphylococcus aureus* in saliva.[18] Risk factors for patients with natural teeth included the preceding 4 or more decayed teeth, number of pairs of opposing teeth, and presence of decay—and periodontal disease-causing organisms in saliva or dental plaque, respectively.

A retrospective analysis of 3 states' Minimum Data Set/Resident Assessment Instrument reports for a 1-year period, representing nearly 103,000 nursing home residents, found the following risk indicators for AP: Chronic obstructive pulmonary disease, congestive heart failure, the use of a feeding tube, bedfast status, high case mix (low functionality/high dependency), delirium, weight loss, swallowing problems, urinary tract infection, mechanical diet, dependence for eating, medical immobility, impaired locomotion, number of medications, and age.[15]

More recently, modifiable risk factors for pneumonia in elderly nursing home residents were identified in a prospective study of 613 elderly residents of 5 nursing homes.[19] In this cohort, 18% developed pneumonia. Statistical modeling suggested that inadequate oral care and difficulty with swallowing were associated with pneumonia.

PATHOGENESIS

Under normal circumstances, the lower airway presents formidable defense against bacteria that are aspirated.[20] A viscous mucous layer coating the epithelium, containing host-derived mucins and antimicrobial components such as lactoperoxidase, lysozyme, and other antimicrobial peptides,[21] traps bacteria, which are then removed from the lung by the mucocutaneous escalator, a function of the unidirectional beating of epithelial cilia. Complex bacterial surface components interact with pattern recognition receptors such as Toll-like receptors to activate inflammation through the nuclear factor-κB signaling pathway. This in turn recruits activated macrophages and neutrophils that engulf the invading bacteria.

Pneumonia is the result of aspiration of infectious agents colonizing the oral cavity and/or upper respiratory tract.[22,23] Any condition that compromises upper airway defenses increases the risk for pneumonia by allowing aspirated bacteria to attach to the respiratory epithelium, which then triggers the cascade of events that result in overt infection (**Fig. 1**). Such conditions include those that reduce containment of the secretions to the upper airway. So, for example, placement of an endotracheal tube through the larynx and trachea into the lung can provide a route for bacteria to bypass those structures that normally prevent aspirations, such as the glottis. Another condition that promotes aspiration is dysphagia, already noted as more common in elderly individuals.[24] Dysphagia is also common in nursing home residents,[25] and therefore represents an important risk factor for AP. Reduction in salivary flow, which occurs frequently in the elderly, most commonly as a side effect of 1 or more medications, also likely contributes to increased risk for pneumonia by allowing enhanced microbial biofilm formation.[26]

It is possible that dysphagia can occur in the absence of overt signs of swallowing difficulty, so-called silent aspiration.[27] Certain conditions, such as stroke or impaired cough reflex, may increase the frequency of such silent aspirations.

In the case of AP, it is likely that most cases are the result of mixed infections involving 2 or more bacterial species, which may be more virulent than infections caused by a single species.[28] Bacteria normally indigenous to the oral cavity can initiate disease, especially anaerobes associated with periodontal disease.[29] Or these species may potentiate the pathogenic potential of other, more typical respiratory pathogens, such as *Streptococcus pneumonia*, *S aureus*, or *Pseudomonas aeruginosa*, which can colonize the oral cavity in high risk subjects such as those in the nursing home.[30,31] It is well documented that potential respiratory pathogens such as *S aureus*, *P aeruginosa*, *Klebsiella pneumoniae*, and *Enterobacter cloacae* colonize the dental plaque of dependent elderly.[32,33] In some health care settings, more than one half the subjects assessed showed the presence of these bacteria in the dental

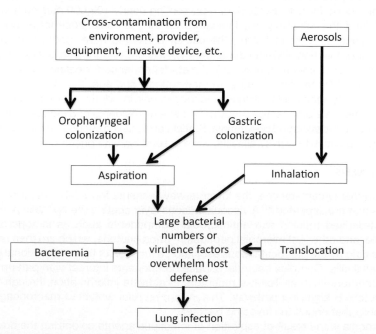

Fig. 1. Factors influencing risk for pneumonia.

plaque, and prevalence of colonization has been correlated with length of time in the setting.[3,23]

ORAL HEALTH AND AP

Before the mid 1990s, the role of oral conditions in the pathogenesis of AP, particularly poor oral hygiene and periodontal inflammation, was mostly ignored in the medical and nursing care setting, although it was understood that the source of the infectious agents causing the disease was often the oral microflora. This situation began to change as knowledge of the specific role of the oral microflora in the pathogenesis of pneumonia became available.[1,23] Much of the work at this time was performed in hospitalized patients, particularly mechanically ventilated patients in the ICU, who have substantially elevated risk for pneumonia. It was shown that the teeth serve as a reservoir for respiratory pathogen colonization,[34–36] and thus serve as a source of bacteria in aspirated secretions. Further studies also suggested that methods to improve oral hygiene in these populations could reduce their risk of pneumonia.[37–39]

Several other studies suggested that the oral cavity might also serve as a reservoir for pulmonary infection in nursing home residents.[32,33,40] Again, the oral cavities of elderly residents of nursing homes were more frequently found to harbor respiratory pathogens than those of ambulatory patients.

There is some evidence that periodontal disease may be associated with risk for pneumonia in elderly patients. A study of an elderly Japanese population found that the adjusted mortality owing to pneumonia was 3.9 times higher in persons with 10 or more teeth with a probing depth exceeding 4 mm (ie, with periodontal pockets) than in those without periodontal pockets.[41]

In light of these findings, it seems intuitively obvious that oral hygiene or periodontal therapy would help to prevent the onset or progression of AP in high-risk patients. Indeed, a number of studies, described herein, have tested this hypothesis.

ORAL CARE TO PREVENT AP

Most of the available literature addressing the role of oral care in the prevention of pneumonia has been conducted in hospitalized and mechanically ventilated patients. However, several studies have also been conducted in nursing home patients. These studies have been critically reviewed in several recent, systematic reviews of the literature. Taken together, the evidence supports the link between poor oral health and pneumonia.[37,42–44] Oral interventions to reduce pulmonary infections have been examined in both mechanically ventilated ICU patients and nonventilated elderly patients.[37,39,42,43] A variety of oral interventions have been tested, including topical antimicrobial agents such as chlorhexidine (CHX) and betadine. Fewer studies have evaluated the effectiveness of traditional oral mechanical hygiene. The use of oral topical CHX reduces pneumonia in mechanically ventilated patients, and may even decrease the need of systemic IV antibiotics or shorten the duration of mechanical ventilation in the ICU.[45–49] Also, oral application of CHX in the early postintubation period lowers the numbers of cultivable oral bacteria and may delay the development of VAP.[50] Not all studies support the effectiveness of oral CHX in reducing pneumonia, however.[51–54] The efficacy of oral CHX decontamination to reduce pneumonia requires further investigation.

Several studies have demonstrated that mechanical oral care, in some cases in combination with povidone iodine, significantly decreases the risk of pneumonia in nursing home residents.[55-57] Once-a-week professional oral cleaning significantly reduced influenza infections in an elderly population.[58]

Implementation of professional oral care programs in nursing facilities involving the deployment of dental hygienists to provide direct oral care, including tooth, tongue, and denture brushing, may help to reduce the oropharyngeal microbial burden, and therefore the number of microbes that can be aspirated into the lower airway.[59] Such an approach may also reduce the risk of other respiratory infections such as influenza.[60]

Oral cleansing reduces pneumonia in both edentulous and dentate subjects, suggesting that oral colonization of bacteria contributes to nosocomial pneumonia to a greater extent than periodontitis per se. However, intervention studies on the treatment of periodontitis on the incidence of pneumonia have not been performed owing to the complexities required in investigating ICU or bed-bound nursing home patients. In edentulous patients, dentures could conceivably serve as a similar reservoir as teeth for oral and respiratory bacterial colonization if not cleaned properly on a daily basis, although neither removable dentures nor the edentulous oral cavity provide the anaerobic environments favored by periodontopathic organisms.

TENTATIVE GUIDELINES FOR ORAL CARE OF DEPENDENT, ELDERLY PATIENTS TO PREVENT RESPIRATORY INFECTION

An important development over the past 10 years has been the establishment of "ventilator bundles," sets of evidence based-therapies instituted within health care settings to reduce the rate of VAP.[61] These bundles include a number of recommended actions, including placement of the patient in a semirecumbent position, stress ulcer prophylaxis to decrease gastrointestinal bleeding, anticoagulant prophylaxis to decrease deep venous thrombosis, adjustment of sedation until the patient can follow commands, and daily assessment of readiness to extubate, to reduce the duration of mechanical ventilation. Implementation of these bundles has been shown to greatly reduce VAP rates.[61] In some cases, oral hygiene care, including topical CHX, has been included as part of the bundles.[62,63]

Paradoxically, the development, validation, and implementation of similar measures focused on preventing NHAP in nursing homes has not occurred even though several studies have demonstrated that improved oral hygiene can reduce the risk of pneumonia in nursing home residents.[64] This is puzzling in that the links between dental, oral, and oropharyngeal colonization by pulmonary pathogens and incidence of AP is based on studies of both ICU and nursing home populations. As such, one would logically expect similar guidance regarding prevention of AP in both settings.

Residents of ICUs are arguably generally less able than nursing home residents to attend to their own daily care needs, owing to the extent of infirmity, altered consciousness, and the presence of physical impediments (eg, ventilator, feeding, and intravenous tubes; restraints). However, individuals are placed in nursing home settings because 1 or more of their essential daily care needs[65] such as bathing (which is usually lumped with all personal hygiene, including mouth care), dressing, transferring, toileting, and eating, cannot be adequately addressed without the services provided in such a facility. For example, the 2004 National Nursing Home Survey[66] reported that 60% to 83% of the approximately 1.5 million Americans residing in nursing homes are extensively or wholly dependent on the assistance of another for addressing their bathing and personal hygiene needs. In contrast with ICU settings, where durations of stay vary from days to weeks, duration of stay in nursing home is generally counted in weeks, months, or years. Unmet daily oral care that is not addressed on behalf of a nursing home resident is likely, over time, to pose a greater threat than the same need in an ICU patient.

Numerous studies have reported on the high prevalence of very poor oral conditions, including inadequate provision of daily oral hygiene, observed in both dentate and edentulous residents of nursing homes.[67,68] Several factors related to nurse education and attitudes toward the significance of oral health to overall well-being contribute to the poor level of oral care in long-term care settings.[69-72] Other, more tangible factors likely play important roles as well. Nurse staffing in ICU settings ranges from 1 nurse per patient to 1 nurse per 3 for patients with lower acuity needs.[73] In contrast with the 8 to 24 hours of nursing care for each ICU patient, residents of nursing homes seldom receive even 3 hours of nurse attention per day and typically receive substantially less,[74] limiting the staff time in the latter setting available for delivering needed cares. ICUs are staffed by registered nurses, whereas the majority of care needs in nursing homes is delivered by nurse aides. Studies have demonstrated strong correlations among nursing home staff between duration of nurse training, income, and the importance accorded to personal as well as patients' oral health. Oral anatomy, oral assessment, and provision of daily oral care are seldom part of nursing curricula, emphasizing the importance of in-service education and on establishing and following protocols, such as the ICU "bundles" described. Nurse aides in long-term care have the highest annual turnover of any clinical position, undermining any potential impact of educational interventions directed to enhancing performance. Finally, the dominant payment sources for ICU services (eg, Medicare and insurance) must ultimately bear the cost of AP, which compels clinical managers to seek out and adopt practices that can prevent onset of the disease. In contrast, the dominant payment source for nursing home care (Medicaid) will not bear the cost for hospitalization owing to AP or even pneumonia care undertaken within the nursing home (Medicare), limiting the impetus for undertaking AP-prevention measures.

A recent paper described clinical practice guidelines for oral hygiene in critically ill patients[75] based on a systematic literature review followed by prospective consideration of the evidence at a consensus development conference. Although there are no rigorous clinical trials that have validated each recommendation, those listed seem reasonable to consider for prevention of AP in frail elderly residents of nursing homes.

1. Systematic clinical assessment of the oral cavity using standardized methods (to include the condition of the teeth, gums, tongue, mucous membranes and lips), upon admission and at least daily thereafter.
2. The use of a soft bristled toothbrush, and dental floss if feasible, to remove debris and dental plaque at least twice a day.
3. The use of mouth swabs (foam and cotton) only when there is a contraindication to brushing (eg, bleeding gums associated with thrombocytopenia).
4. The use of 1 oral rinse over another was considered questionable (with the exception of chlorhexidine gluconate 0.12% in the cardiac surgical patients).
5. Although the optimal duration for oral care focused on reducing risk of AP has not been determined, oral cleansing for 3 to 4 minutes using a brush that allows access to all areas of the mouth was suggested.

SUMMARY

Understanding the risk factors and preventive measures for AP is essential in the care of hospitalized and institutionalized, disabled elderly. Control of oral biofilm formation in these populations reduces the numbers of potential respiratory pathogens in the oral secretions, which in turn reduces the risk for pneumonia. Together with other preventive measures (head of the bed position, promotion of salivary flow, vaccination against pathogens such as *S pneumoniae*, management of swallowing disorders, etc), improved oral hygiene helps to control lower respiratory infections in frail elderly hospital and nursing home patients.

REFERENCES

1. Raghavendran K, Mylotte JM, Scannapieco FA. Nursing home-associated pneumonia, hospital-acquired pneumonia and ventilator-associated pneumonia: the contribution of dental biofilms and periodontal inflammation. Periodontol 2000 2007;44:164–77.
2. Marik PE. Aspiration pneumonitis and aspiration pneumonia. N Engl J Med 2001;344(9):665–71.
3. Shay K, Scannapieco FA, Terpenning MS, et al. Nosocomial pneumonia and oral health. Spec Care Dentist 2005;25(4):179–87.
4. Hoyert DL, Xu J. Deaths: preliminary data for 2011. Natl Vital Stat Rep 2012; 61(6):1–7.
5. Yende S, Alvarez K, Loehr L, et al. Epidemiology and long-term clinical and biologic risk factors for pneumonia in community-dwelling older Americans: analysis of three cohorts. Chest 2013;144(3):1008–17.
6. Flanders SA, Collard HR, Saint S. Nosocomial pneumonia: state of the science. Am J Infect Control 2006;34(2):84–93.
7. Medina-Walpole AM, Katz PR. Nursing home-acquired pneumonia. J Am Geriatr Soc 1999;47(8):1005–15.
8. Tablan OC, Anderson LJ, Besser R, et al. Guidelines for preventing health-care–associated pneumonia, 2003: recommendations of CDC and the Healthcare Infection Control Practices Advisory Committee. MMWR Recomm Rep 2004; 53(RR-3):1–36.
9. Mylotte JM. Nursing home-acquired pneumonia. Clin Infect Dis 2002;35(10): 1205–11.
10. Muder RR. Pneumonia in residents of long-term care facilities: epidemiology, etiology, management, and prevention. Am J Med 1998;105(4):319–30.
11. Mylotte JM. Nursing home-associated pneumonia. Clin Geriatr Med 2007;23(3): 553–65, vi–vii.
12. Dosa D. Should I hospitalize my resident with nursing home-acquired pneumonia? J Am Med Dir Assoc 2006;7(Suppl 3):S74–80, 73.
13. Vincent JL, Bihari DJ, Suter PM, et al. The prevalence of nosocomial infection in intensive care units in Europe. Results of the European Prevalence of Infection in Intensive Care (EPIC) study. EPIC International Advisory Committee. JAMA 1995;274(8):639–44.
14. Marik PE, Kaplan D. Aspiration pneumonia and dysphagia in the elderly. Chest 2003;124(1):328–36.
15. Langmore SE, Skarupski KA, Park PS, et al. Predictors of aspiration pneumonia in nursing home residents. Dysphagia 2002;17(4):298–307.
16. van der Maarel-Wierink CD, Vanobbergen JN, Bronkhorst EM, et al. Meta-analysis of dysphagia and aspiration pneumonia in frail elders. J Dent Res 2011; 90(12):1398–404.
17. Langmore SE, Terpenning MS, Schork A, et al. Predictors of aspiration pneumonia: how important is dysphagia? Dysphagia 1998;13:69–81.

18. Terpenning MS, Taylor GW, Lopatin DE, et al. Aspiration pneumonia: dental and oral risk factors in an older veteran population. J Am Geriatr Soc 2001;49:557–63.
19. Quagliarello V, Ginter S, Han L, et al. Modifiable risk factors for nursing home-acquired pneumonia. Clin Infect Dis 2005;40(1):1–6.
20. Gellatly SL, Hancock RE. *Pseudomonas aeruginosa*: new insights into pathogenesis and host defenses. Pathog Dis 2013;67(3):159–73.
21. Gerson C, Sabater J, Scuri M, et al. The lactoperoxidase system functions in bacterial clearance of airways. Am J Respir Cell Mol Biol 2000;22(6):665–71.
22. Johanson WG, Dever LL. Nosocomial pneumonia. Intensive Care Med 2003; 29(1):23–9.
23. Scannapieco FA. Role of oral bacteria in respiratory infection. J Periodontol 1999;70(7):793–802.
24. Sue Eisenstadt E. Dysphagia and aspiration pneumonia in older adults. J Am Acad Nurse Pract 2010;22(1):17–22.
25. Park YH, Han HR, Oh BM, et al. Prevalence and associated factors of dysphagia in nursing home residents. Geriatr Nurs 2013;34(3):212–7.
26. Gupta A, Epstein JB, Sroussi H. Hyposalivation in elderly patients. J Can Dent Assoc 2006;72(9):841–6.
27. Ramsey D, Smithard D, Kalra L. Silent aspiration: what do we know? Dysphagia 2005;20(3):218–25.
28. Kimizuka R, Kato T, Ishihara K, et al. Mixed infections with *Porphyromonas gingivalis* and *Treponema denticola* cause excessive inflammatory responses in a mouse pneumonia model compared with monoinfections. Microbes Infect 2003; 5(15):1357–62.
29. Bartlett JG. Anaerobic bacterial infection of the lung. Anaerobe 2012;18(2): 235–9.
30. Pan Y, Teng D, Burke AC, et al. Oral bacteria modulate invasion and induction of apoptosis in HEp-2 cells by *Pseudomonas aeruginosa*. Microb Pathog 2009; 46(2):73–9.
31. Li Q, Pan C, Teng D, et al. Porphyromonas gingivalis modulates *Pseudomonas aeruginosa*-induced apoptosis of respiratory epithelial cells through the STAT3 signaling pathway. Microbes Infect 2014;16(1):17–27.
32. Russell SL, Boylan RJ, Kaslick RS, et al. Respiratory pathogen colonization of the dental plaque of institutionalized elders. Spec Care Dentist 1999;19(3):128–34.
33. Sumi Y, Miura H, Michiwaki Y, et al. Colonization of dental plaque by respiratory pathogens in dependent elderly. Arch Gerontol Geriatr 2007;44(2):119–24.
34. Scannapieco FA, Stewart EM, Mylotte JM. Colonization of dental plaque by respiratory pathogens in medical intensive care patients. Crit Care Med 1992;20(6): 740–5.
35. El-Solh AA, Pietrantoni C, Bhat A, et al. Colonization of dental plaques: a reservoir of respiratory pathogens for hospital-acquired pneumonia in institutionalized elders. Chest 2004;126(5):1575–82.
36. Heo SM, Haase EM, Lesse AJ, et al. Genetic relationships between respiratory pathogens isolated from dental plaque and bronchoalveolar lavage fluid from patients in the intensive care unit undergoing mechanical ventilation. Clin Infect Dis 2008;47(12):1562–70.
37. Azarpazhooh A, Leake JL. Systematic review of the association between respiratory diseases and oral health. J Periodontol 2006;77(9):1465–82.
38. Labeau SO, Van de Vyver K, Brusselaers N, et al. Prevention of ventilator-associated pneumonia with oral antiseptics: a systematic review and meta-analysis. Lancet Infect Dis 2011;11(11):845–54.

39. Shi Z, Xie H, Wang P, et al. Oral hygiene care for critically ill patients to prevent ventilator-associated pneumonia. Cochrane Database Syst Rev 2013;(8): CD008367.

40. Didilescu AC, Skaug N, Marica C, et al. Respiratory pathogens in dental plaque of hospitalized patients with chronic lung diseases. Clin Oral Investig 2005;9(3): 141–7.

41. Awano S, Ansai T, Takata Y, et al. Oral health and mortality risk from pneumonia in the elderly. J Dent Res 2008;87(4):334–9.

42. Scannapieco FA, Bush RB, Paju S. Associations between periodontal disease and risk for nosocomial bacterial pneumonia and chronic obstructive pulmonary disease. A systematic review. Ann Periodontol 2003;8(1):54–69.

43. Chan EY, Ruest A, Meade MO, et al. Oral decontamination for prevention of pneumonia in mechanically ventilated adults: systematic review and meta-analysis. BMJ 2007;334(7599):889.

44. Roberts N, Moule P. Chlorhexidine and tooth-brushing as prevention strategies in reducing ventilator-associated pneumonia rates. Nurs Crit Care 2011;16(6): 295–302.

45. DeRiso AJ 2nd, Ladowski JS, Dillon TA, et al. Chlorhexidine gluconate 0.12% oral rinse reduces the incidence of total nosocomial respiratory infection and nonprophylactic systemic antibiotic use in patients undergoing heart surgery. Chest 1996;109(6):1556–61.

46. Genuit T, Bochicchio G, Napolitano LM, et al. Prophylactic chlorhexidine oral rinse decreases ventilator-associated pneumonia in surgical ICU patients. Surg Infect (Larchmt) 2001;2(1):5–18.

47. Fourrier F, Cau-Pottier E, Boutigny H, et al. Effects of dental plaque antiseptic decontamination on bacterial colonization and nosocomial infections in critically ill patients. Intensive Care Med 2000;26(9):1239–47.

48. Koeman M, van der Ven AJ, Hak E, et al. Oral decontamination with chlorhexidine reduces the incidence of ventilator-associated pneumonia. Am J Respir Crit Care Med 2006;173(12):1348–55.

49. Munro CL, Grap MJ, Jones DJ, et al. Chlorhexidine, toothbrushing, and preventing ventilator-associated pneumonia in critically ill adults. Am J Crit Care 2009; 18(5):428–37 [quiz: 38].

50. Grap MJ, Munro CL, Elswick RK Jr, et al. Duration of action of a single, early oral application of chlorhexidine on oral microbial flora in mechanically ventilated patients: a pilot study. Heart Lung 2004;33(2):83–91.

51. Fourrier F, Dubois D, Pronnier P, et al. Effect of gingival and dental plaque antiseptic decontamination on nosocomial infections acquired in the intensive care unit: a double-blind placebo-controlled multicenter study. Crit Care Med 2005; 33(8):1728–35.

52. Houston S, Hougland P, Anderson JJ, et al. Effectiveness of 0.12% chlorhexidine gluconate oral rinse in reducing prevalence of nosocomial pneumonia in patients undergoing heart surgery. Am J Crit Care 2002;11(6):567–70.

53. Panchabhai TS, Dangayach NS, Krishnan A, et al. Oropharyngeal cleansing with 0.2% chlorhexidine for prevention of nosocomial pneumonia in critically ill patients: an open-label randomized trial with 0.01% potassium permanganate as control. Chest 2009;135(5):1150–6.

54. Scannapieco FA, Yu J, Raghavendran K, et al. A randomized trial of chlorhexidine gluconate on oral bacterial pathogens in mechanically ventilated patients. Crit Care 2009;13(4):R117.

55. Adachi M, Ishihara K, Abe S, et al. Effect of professional oral health care on the elderly living in nursing homes. Oral Surg Oral Med Oral Pathol Oral Radiol Endod 2002;94(2):191–5.

56. Yoneyama T, Hashimoto K, Fukuda H, et al. Oral hygiene reduces respiratory infections in elderly bed-bound nursing home patients. Arch Gerontol Geriatr 1996;22:11–9.

57. Yoneyama T, Yoshida M, Ohrui T, et al. Oral care reduces pneumonia in older patients in nursing homes. J Am Geriatr Soc 2002;50(3):430–3.

58. Molloy J, Wolff LF, Lopez-Guzman A, et al. The association of periodontal disease parameters with systemic medical conditions and tobacco use. J Clin Periodontol 2004;31(8):625–32.

59. Ishikawa A, Yoneyama T, Hirota K, et al. Professional oral health care reduces the number of oropharyngeal bacteria. J Dent Res 2008;87(6):594–8.

60. Abe S, Ishihara K, Adachi M, et al. Professional oral care reduces influenza infection in elderly. Arch Gerontol Geriatr 2006;43(2):157–64.

61. Berenholtz SM, Pham JC, Thompson DA, et al. Collaborative cohort study of an intervention to reduce ventilator-associated pneumonia in the intensive care unit. Infect Control Hosp Epidemiol 2011;32(4):305–14.

62. Caserta RA, Marra AR, Durao MS, et al. A program for sustained improvement in preventing ventilator associated pneumonia in an intensive care setting. BMC Infect Dis 2012;12:234.

63. Eom JS, Lee MS, Chun HK, et al. The impact of a ventilator bundle on preventing ventilator-associated pneumonia: a multicenter study. Am J Infect Control 2013; 42(1):34–7.

64. Sjogren P, Nilsson E, Forsell M, et al. A systematic review of the preventive effect of oral hygiene on pneumonia and respiratory tract infection in elderly people in hospitals and nursing homes: effect estimates and methodological quality of randomized controlled trials. J Am Geriatr Soc 2008;56(11):2124–30.

65. Katz S, Downs TD, Cash HR, et al. Progress in development of the index of ADL. Gerontologist 1970;10(1):20–30.

66. Jones AL, Dwyer LL, Bercovitz AR, et al. The National Nursing Home Survey: 2004 overview. Vital Health Stat 13 2009;(167):1–155.

67. Berkey DB, Berg RG, Ettinger DL, et al. Research review of oral health status and service use among institutionalized older adults in the United States and Canada. Spec Care Dentist 1991;11:131–6.

68. Kiyak HA, Grayston MN, Crinean CL. Oral health problems and needs of nursing home residents. Community Dent Oral Epidemiol 1993;21:49–52.

69. Chalmers JM, Levy SM, Buckwalter KC, et al. Factors influencing nurses' aides' provision of oral care for nursing facility residents. Spec Care Dentist 1996;16(2):71–9.

70. Wardh I, Andersson L, Sorensen S. Staff attitudes to oral health care. A comparative study of registered nurses, nursing assistants and home care aides. Gerodontology 1997;14(1):28–32.

71. Frenkel HF. Behind the screens: care staff observations on delivery of oral health care in nursing homes. Gerodontology 1999;16(2):75–80.

72. Chung JP, Mojon P, Budtz-Jorgensen E. Dental care of elderly in nursing homes: perceptions of managers, nurses, and physicians. Spec Care Dentist 2000; 20(1):12–7.

73. Harrington C, Olney B, Carrillo H, et al. Nurse staffing and deficiencies in the largest for-profit nursing home chains and chains owned by private equity companies. Health Serv Res 2012;47(1 Pt 1):106–28.

74. Hartigan RC. The Synergy Model. Establishing criteria for 1:1 staffing ratios. Crit Care Nurse 2000;20(2):112, 114–6.

75. Berry AM, Davidson PM, Nicholson L, et al. Consensus based clinical guideline for oral hygiene in the critically ill. Intensive Crit Care Nurs 2011;27(4): 180–5.

Oral Implications of Polypharmacy in the Elderly

Mabi L. Singh, DMD, MS[a,b,*], Athena Papas, DMD, PhD[b]

KEYWORDS

- Saliva • Medications • Salivary hypofunction • Elderly • Polypharmacy

KEY POINTS

- The elderly population is increasing and has the highest number of users of prescription and over-the-counter (OTC) medication.
- Age-related changes occur in the body, which affect pharmacokinetics and pharmacodynamics.
- Prescription and OTC medications can cause myriad side effects in the oral cavity, and the elderly are more vulnerable.
- The adverse events in the oral cavity may cause discomfort and loss of function and decrease quality of life in the elderly.

INTRODUCTION

Early diagnoses and treatment of diseases have led to longer life expectancy. However, the treatments of these diseases involve pharmacologic agents, and as people age, they develop multiple health ailments, which can lead to polypharmacy. There are age-related changes in the systems of the body, which alter the pharmacokinetics and pharmacodynamics of medications and make the elderly more vulnerable to adverse events. A major side effects of medications is the qualitative and quantitative change the cause in saliva (salivary hypofunction), by their anticholinergic effects. Saliva plays a pivotal role in the homeostasis of the oral cavity because of its protective and

Funding sources: Invado Pharmeceuticals Grant.

Conflict of interest: none.

[a] Dry Mouth Clinic, Tufts University School of Dental Medicine, 1 Kneeland Street, Boston, MA 02111, USA; [b] Division of Oral Medicine, Department of Oral Pathology, Oral Medicine, Craniofacial Pain, Tufts University School of Dental Medicine, 1 Kneeland Street, Boston, MA 02111, USA

* Corresponding author. Department of Oral Pathology, Oral Medicine, Craniofacial Pain Center, Tufts University School of Dental Medicine, 1 Kneeland Street, Boston, MA 02111.

E-mail address: Mabi_l.singh@tufts.edu

functional properties, which include facilitating speech, swallowing, enhancing taste, buffering and neutralizing intrinsic and extrinsic acid, remineralizing teeth, maintaining the oral mucosal health, preventing overgrowth of noxious microorganisms and xerostomia. With salivary hypofunction, a plethora of complications arise, resulting in decreased quality of life in the elderly. However, the anticholinergic effects of medications can be overcome, and the oral cavity can be restored to normalcy.

CHANGES IN THE ELDERLY POPULATION

With improvements in health care, nutrition, lifestyles, habits, and safety practices, the life expectancy of people in the United States is increasing. This trend is true regardless of race or sex. From 1950 to 2010, the life expectancy of Americans of all races, both male and female, rose from 68.2 years to 78.7 years. The average life expectancy for white Americans (78.9 years) is longer than that of black or African Americans (75.1 years). Further, the life expectancy of white women is 81.3 years, compared with that of white men at 76.5 years. The life expectancy of black women is also longer than that of black men, at 78 years and 71.8 years, respectively.[1]

Globally, with the increase in life expectancy, the demographics of the total population are changing. In 2011, 14% of the total population of the United States was older than 65 years. It is estimated that in 2020, this percentage will increase to 16.76%, and by 2050, the percentage of people, both male and female, older than 65 years in the total population will increase to 20.95%.[2]

AGE-RELATED EFFECTS ON THE BODY

Chronologic aging is a process that affects various biological and physiologic processes in the human body. With advancing age, the functional abilities of organ systems tend to decrease. Although there is variability in the age-related changes that take place within each individual, aging generally affects all of the major biological and physiologic systems of the body.

For example, as one ages, there is a change in the composition of the body leading to a decrease in total body water and lean body mass, countered by an increase in body fat. Together, these age-related changes result in a diminished ability to distribute, metabolize, and excrete (clear) certain drugs. This situation causes water-soluble medications to be processed differently and less effectively. Lipophilic drugs because they have an increased volume of distribution, causing a prolonged half life, whereas water-soluble drugs have a smaller volume of distribution and a shorter half life.[3]

The liver is affected in several ways as the body ages. Specifically, there is a decrease in hepatic mass, hepatic blood flow, and enzymatic efficiency. The kidneys also undergo age-related alterations, such as a decrease in renal plasma flow, glomerular filtration rate, and tubular secretion. After these changes, as one ages, there is an increased sensitivity to medications, which can result in medication-induced hepatotoxicity and nephrotoxicity. In the cardiovascular system, the elasticity of blood vessels begins to decrease with age. This stiffening of blood vessels results in the decreased mechanical effectiveness of the heart. Furthermore, in the gastrointestinal system, the secretion of hydrochloric acid and pepsin decreases with the aging of the body. This situation then results in changes in absorption in the gastrointestinal tract.[4]

In the salivary glands, the aging process may cause the number of acinar cells to be reduced and to be replaced by fibrous and fatty tissue. This process may cause the composition of saliva to change.[5–7]

THE ELDERLY AND MEDICATIONS

The elderly population is more susceptible to acute and chronic medical problems. Hence, to cure or treat the ailments, either prescription medications or nonprescription (over-the-counter [OTC]) medications are introduced in the body system. In 2007 to 2008, more than 88% of Americans older than 60 years took at least 1 prescription medication, 76% used 2 or more prescription medications, and 37% used 5 or more. The use of at least 1 prescription medication follows a linear trend as the aging process advances. This trend is different in men and women, with women using more prescription drugs than men. Significantly more non-Hispanic whites take medications than non-Hispanic blacks or Mexican Americans. Even although the elderly represent only 13% of the population, one-third of the prescriptions written are dispensed to this population.[8]

In addition, as more prescription medications are being changed to OTC status, increasingly older adults self-manage medications to treat common medical conditions, especially the common cold, pain, diarrhea, constipation, indigestion, and headache.[9] Surveys[10] indicate that the elderly use 2 to 4 nonprescription medications daily, most commonly nonsteroidal antiinflammatory drugs, antihistamines, antacids (H_2 blockers), laxatives, and sedatives.[11]

Also, the increased use of illicit drugs by senior has become an emerging issue which prompted the National Institutes of Health to circulate an alert in 2012 about improper use of substances, to strengthen public awareness of substance use disorders in the elderly.[12]

Most Common Anticholinergic Medications

The most common anticholinergic medications are listed in **Table 1**.

Side Effects of Medications

Apart from their therapeutic effect, pharmacologic agents also bind to other unwanted potential sites causing side effects that affect the central nervous system (CNS) and/or the peripheral nervous system. Central side effects include confusion/disorientation, hallucinations, sleepiness, clumsiness or unsteadiness, convulsions, mental status/behavior changes such as distress, excitement, nervousness, attention deficits, cognitive decline (memory loss), and delirium. Peripheral side effects of medications can be salivary hypofunction, difficulty in speech and swallowing, mucous membrane dryness of the nose and skin, blurred vision, light sensitivity, increased breathing difficulty, difficulty urinating, bloating, and constipation in older adults.[13,14]

The perception of dry mouth has been reported to be directly proportional to the total number of drugs taken per day. Dry.org reports 1800 drugs in 80 drug classes that have the capacity to induce xerostomia.[15] Because there are more new medications in the pipeline in production to cure and treat diseases, the list of salivary hypofunction-inducing medications will only increase.

How Does Anticholinergic Medication Work?

To achieve therapeutic benefits and manage diseases, medications with anticholinergic properties are used. Anticholinergic medications competitively block or prevent acetylcholine molecules, which are neurotransmitters, from adhering to receptors of the cell membrane in both the central and peripheral nervous systems. Molecular cloning has defined 5 distinct muscarinic cholinergic receptor subtypes, designated M_1 to M_5, with each subtype being encoded by distinct cellular genes.[16]

Table 1
Common medications with significant anticholinergic properties and potential adverse consequences

Indication	Drug
First-generation antihistamines (as single agent or as part of combination products)	Chlorpheniramine Cyproheptadine Brompheniramine Carbinoxamine Chlorpheniramine Clemastine Cyproheptadine Dexbrompheniramine Diphenhydramine (oral) Doxylamine Hydroxyzine Promethazine Triprolidine

Antidepressants
SSRI and SNRI
	SSRI
	  Fluoxetine
	  Paroxetine
	  Sertraline
	  Fluvoxamine
	  Citalopram
	SNRI
	  Venlafaxine
	  Duloxetine
	  Desvenlafaxine

Antidiarrheal	Diphenoxylate atropine
Anti-Parkinson	Amantadine benztropine Biperiden trihexyphenidyl
Muscle relaxants	Cyclobenzaprine dantrolene Orphenadrine
Antivertigo	Meclizine scopolamine Phenothiazine
Tricyclic antidepressants, alone or in combination	Amitriptyline Chlordiazepoxide-amitriptyline Clomipramine Doxepin Imipramine Perphenazine Trimipramine
Cardiovascular	Furosemide Digoxin Nifedipine Disopyramide
Antispasmodic medications	Belladonna alkaloids Clidinium–chlordiazepoxide Dicyclomine Hyoscyamine Propantheline Scopolamine
Antiulcer	Cimetidine ranitidine
Antipsychotic	Chlorpromazine clozapine Olanzapine thioridazine Mesoridazine
Urinary incontinence	Oxybutynin probantheline Solifenacin tolterodine Trospium
Antiemetics	Prochlorperazine promethazine

Adapted from Minnesota Department of Health. Available at: http://www.health.state.mn.us/divs/fpc/cww/D02_Transmittal22ExcerptTableII.pdf Accessed January 1, 2014; and American Geriatrics Society Beers criteria for potentially inappropriate medication use in older adults. Available at: http://www.americangeriatrics.org/files/documents/beers/PrintableBeersPocketCard.pdf Accessed January 1, 2014.

M_3 receptors are found in the CNS, airway smooth muscles, and glandular tissues (such as salivary gland tissue). When the anticholinergics adhere to the receptors, especially on the M_3 receptors of the salivary gland, cell membrane changes are prevented (like the inhibition of adenylate cyclase, or the alteration in calcium permeability that leads to cholinergic responses).[17] When multiple medications are being taken at the same time for the treatments of various ailments of the elderly, their anticholinergic properties are potentiated. The cumulative anticholinergic burden of multiple medications and metabolites, rather than of a single compound causes the toxicities that are seen in the elderly.[18] Each year, adverse drug events affect millions causing considerable morbidity and mortality.[19]

Anticholinergic agents compete with the muscarinic receptors in the salivary glands and alter their function, but do not interact with or prevent the formation of acetylcholine.

Beers criteria

Mark Beers, MD, a geriatrician, created the Beers criteria which catalogs medications that cause adverse drug events in older adults because of their pharmacologic properties and/or the physiologic changes of aging. In 2011, the American Geriatrics Society (AGS) updated the criteria, assembling a team of experts, using an enhanced, evidence-based methodology. Each criterion is rated using the American College of Physicians' Guideline Grading system, which is based on the Grading of Recommendations Assessment, Development and Evaluation (GRADE) developed by Guyatt and colleagues.[20]

ROLE OF SALIVA

Saliva is produced by 3 pairs of major salivary glands and 400 to 600 minor salivary glands. The serous (watery) portion of the saliva is mostly produced by the parotid and submandibular (mixed serous and mucous) glands, and the mucus (mucin-containing) part is produced by the submandibular, sublingual, and minor salivary glands. Ninety-five percent of the saliva is produced by the salivary glands. The rate of whole unstimulated salivary flow is about 0.3 mL/min (average), and stimulated is on average 1.5 mL/min (with large individual variability). The critical level of saliva is considered to be less than between 0.1 and 0.16 mL/min when the complications from the salivary hypofunction arise.[21,22] Bicarbonates, Sialin, ammonia, urea and water in saliva buffer and neutralize the intrinsic and extrinsic acid and restore the normal pH in the oral cavity. Because of lubricating actions, saliva is necessary for speech, the bolus formation, and swallowing. Saliva also aids in flushing away food debris, dead tissue, and biofilm. Antimicrobial proteins and peptides in saliva (eg, histatins, lysozyme, lactoperoxidase, and lactoferrin) keep the deleterious microorganisms in check in the microenvironment of the oral cavity.[23]

Because secretory salivary IgA and mucins are reduced in the healthy elderly, the oral soft tissues become more susceptible to environmental factors as a result of a reduction of both immunologic and nonimmunologic defense systems of the oral cavity.[24]

ADVERSE EVENTS OF SALIVARY HYPOFUNCTION IN THE ORAL CAVITY

The peripheral side effects of anticholinergic drugs can lead to a plethora of dental and oral complications. Some of the common complications are listed later. The Anticholinergic Risk Scale (ARS) is useful tool that helps to assess the risk of adverse effects caused by anticholinergic drugs. Within the scale, medications are categorized with, each category being assigned points. To use the ARS, the points are added up with the higher the total points, having the greater the risk.[25]

Xerostomia

The subjective sensation of dryness in the oral cavity is called xerostomia.[26] The aging process may cause the number of acinar cells to be reduced and to be replaced by fibrous and fatty tissue, but the composition remains the same in nonmedicated elders. Xerostomia is not a natural consequence of aging, but its prevalence increases with age.[27] When the basal volume of unstimulated saliva, which usually coats the soft and hard tissue, is decreased by 50% to 70% of the original volume, the subjective sensation of dryness occurs, resulting in xerostomia. Initially, the serous portion of the whole saliva is lost, leaving primarily the mucous portion. Consequently, secretion of thick and viscous saliva leads to a perception of having excessive saliva in the oral cavity. The anticholinergic load of drug(s) determines the severity of the reduction of salivary production that leads to xerostomia. It is more prevalent in the elderly population, primarily because of their increased use of drugs and their susceptibility to disease. Many drugs and drug classes have been linked to xerostomia; the xerogenic effect increases with poly pharmacy.[28]

Dental Carious Lesions

Just like bone, teeth are mineralized tissues that constantly undergo demineralization and remineralization controlled by saliva.[29] Saliva is normally supersaturated with calcium and phosphate ions acid either extrinsic or intrinsic leaches mineral from teeth. Fluoride acts as a catalyst to promote remineralization and is incorporated in the crystal to create a harder less soluble tooth structure, thus maintaining homeostasis in the oral cavity.

In salivary hypofunction, because of a decreased quantity of saliva and the loss of the antimicrobial functions of saliva, the number of cariogenic microorganisms (*Streptococcus mutans* lactobacilli) and *Candida* increases. In addition, the food (carbohydrate) substrate and dead cells are no longer debrided/lavaged well, thereby providing more substrate from which microorganisms produce bacterial acid to demineralize the tooth structure. Also, the loss of saliva enhances aggregation and adherence of noxious microorganisms, resulting in an increased population of bacteria. Normally, the demineralized structures are remineralized, but in the compromised microenvironment of the oral cavity, the potential to remineralize is decreased, thus increasing the risk of developing new and recurrent carious lesions. With elderly Americans living longer, retaining their teeth longer, resulting in a significant reduction in edentulism. With this change, along with receding gingival levels, more root surfaces are exposed, leading to an increased surface at risk (SAR) (**Figs. 1** and **2**). More than half of the individuals older than 65 years have experienced root caries.[30]

Candidiasis

The decrease in qualitative and quantitative saliva disposes to oral candidiasis. Studies have found the presence of *Candida* spp in association with mutans streptococci and lactobacilli in the saliva associated with dental decay and decreased microhardness of enamel.[31,32] In patients with oral candidiasis, salivary levels of lactoferrin, secretory immunoglobulins, salivary proteins, and peptides may be decreased and give rise to the growth and adhesion of candidial species to the oral tissue. Fissuring of the tongue, denture prosthesis, the presence of other (autoimmune) diseases affecting salivary gland function, and oral hygiene habits can increase aggregation, adherence, and penetration into deeper tissues and subsequently increase the risk of candidiasis.

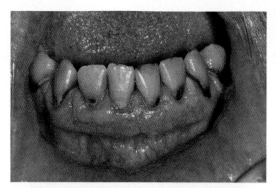

Fig. 1. In older adults, more root surfaces are exposed, leading to an increased SAR.

When the opportunistic candidial microorganisms overgrow on the mucosa of the oral cavity, it may present with no obvious clinical presentation or present as erythematous, pseudomembranous, hyperplastic or angular chelitis. In salivary hypofunction, even the dental prostheses in the oral cavity can provide additional surfaces for the adherence and growth of the candidial population (**Fig. 3**).

Burning Tongue

Loss of the lubricating function of saliva may lead to increased friction between the tongue and hard tissue in the oral cavity. Candidiasis, fissuring of the tongue, sensitivity to allergens, strong tastants, and supertaster status can contribute to the burning sensation of the tongue.

Tooth Surface Loss

Tooth surface loss and caries are due to the irreversible loss of the tooth minerals. Enamel dissolves at the critical pH of 5.8 and dentin at 6.9. In the presence of fluoride, tooth structure is remineralized with the formation of hydroxyfluoroapatite crystals, but frequent acid exposures tips the balance to demineralization, resulting in caries, erosion, abrasion, and attrition.

Saliva is the most critical biological factor to prevent erosion. In the absence of the buffering action of saliva, there is a decreased potential of forming a pellicle (a protective barrier to the hard tissue), which helps prevent the direct exposure of the teeth to

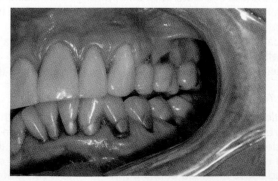

Fig. 2. In older adults, more root surfaces are exposed, leading to an increased SAR.

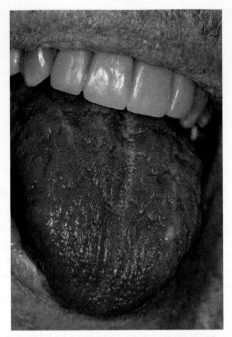

Fig. 3. In salivary hypofunction, even the dental prostheses in the oral cavity can provide additional surfaces for the adherence and growth of the candidial population.

extrinsic and intrinsic acidic challenges in the oral cavity. Erosive lesions follow. There occurs a characteristic cupping or saucerlike appearance of the cuspal tips and incisal edges, a thinning of enamel, and subsequent yellowing of teeth. Lesions in which the width is greater than the depth, with loss of luster and matted look, can be found on the smooth surfaces, resulting from the process of erosion. Because of tooth surface loss around restorations, restorations may look as though they are protruding out of the tooth surfaces. These restorations are called proud restorations.

Also, because of a lack of lubricating action of saliva, tooth to tooth mechanical contact can result in tooth surface loss, called attrition. Tooth attrition takes place during the physiologic aging process, usually resulting in the loss of vertical height of the tooth. In the elderly cohort with salivary hypofunction, attrition can be accentuated, especially if the hardness of a restoration on opposing teeth is different than the tooth structure and pathologic. The vertical occlusal forces can result in the attrition of the incisal edges and abfraction of cervical and proximal surfaces.

The mechanical forces including chewing, deglutition, and parafunctional habits, cause wear facets, which are usually flat and well circumscribed in both opposing arches. Once the attrition reaches the dentin, the loss accelerates (**Fig. 4**).[33]

Fissuring of the Tongue

Aging and genetic predisposition can lead to central furrowing, with lateral extension of the dorsal surface of tongue, with varied depths. Salivary mucins protect the oral cavity against desiccation and environmental insult by coating the mucosal surfaces.[34] Loss of natural protective and environmental factors can cause fissuring of the tongue. Dead tissue and food debris trapped inside these grooves can serve as a feeding and breeding ground for biofilm and cause inflammation and halitosis.

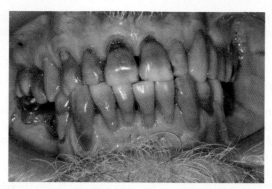

Fig. 4. Once the attrition reaches the dentin, the loss of the tooth structure can be rapid.

Because removal of debris and biofilm from the deeper and fissured tongue is difficult, development of biofilm on other parts of the oral structures may be accelerated. Irritation of exposed or nearly exposed nerve endings on the cracked mucosal lining may induce increased sensitivity to tastants and other particles (**Fig. 5**).

Difficulty with Swallowing and Speech

The quantitative and qualitative decrease in saliva interferes with speech and swallowing processes as a result of loss of lubrication and decreased capability to form a bolus.

Mucositis

The oral mucosa is vulnerable to inflammation and ulceration because of cells in the process of mitosis, exposure to foreign objects, and reduced functioning of saliva. The mucositis can be accentuated by sharp dental edges, faulty restorations, or ill-fitting dentures.

Loss of Taste Perception

Decreased transfer of tastants by saliva to the receptor cells of the taste buds of the gustatory system, as well as possible coating of the tongue, as a result of microbial growth and accumulation of dead tissue and food debris, may interfere with the taste perception. Taste perception may be exaggerated if denuding of the tongue occurs as

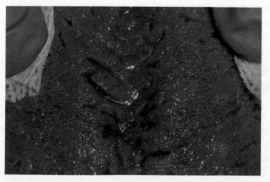

Fig. 5. Irritation of exposed or nearly exposed nerve endings on the cracked mucosal lining may induce increased sensitivity to tastants and other particles.

a result of loss of partial or total loss of papillae or alteration of the papillary architecture. Also, depending on type of medication use, there may be altered taste (eg, a metallic taste).

OVERCOMING ANTICHOLINERGIC EFFECTS

In contrast to the irreversible salivary hypofunction caused by Sjögren's syndrome and the therapeutic radiation of the head and neck area, medications and their side effects cause no physical damage to the salivary gland cells. Both gustatory or mechanical stimulation of the salivary glands promotes salivary flow.

As competitive antagonists, the effect of anticholinergic drugs can be overcome by increasing the concentration of acetylcholine in muscarinic M_3 receptors and increase production of saliva from the salivary glands. The anticholinergics may also cause vasodilation, acid production, and bronchodilatation. Parasympathomimetic drugs (eg, pilocarpine HCl [nonselective muscarinic agonist] and cevimeline HCl [M_1 and M_3 selectivity]), can bind with M_3 receptors and increase the intracellular Ca^{2+} concentration in salivary acini. Also, pilocarpine can increase the blood flow with the pressor response (due to increase in arterial pressure).[35] The stimulatory action of pilocarpine and cevimiline lasts up to 3 hours and 5 hours, respectively. Cevimiline induces salivary secretion at higher doses (30 mg) compared with pilocarpine (5 mg). Cevimeline may have lower sensitivity to Ca^{2+} in salivary glands[36,37] and be less effective in the heart and lungs with M_2 and M_4 muscarinic receptors.

Because of unwanted therapeutic effects of sialogogues, with individual variability, the dosage should be titrated up to the maximum and given for as long as 3 months for full effect.

MECHANICAL AND GUSTATORY STIMULATION

Gustatory and mechanical actions in the oral cavity, via neural reflexes, stimulate saliva, which increases the buffering capability, pH, and supersaturation of the salivary minerals (eg, calcium and phosphate).

Chewing sugar-free gum over a prolonged period results in a functional increase in salivary flow, as well as in increases in pH and buffer capacity which can help reduce plaque acidogenicity.[38] In a Cochrane review,[39] chewing gums increased saliva production in those with residual secretory capacity and was preferred by patients.

Also, manual (massaging) and thermal (moist heat) stimulation of parotid and submandibular glands helps expel mucous plugs and small sialoliths, which may cause salivary gland swelling and damage.

XYLITOL

The effects of xylitol-incorporated lozenges, spray, and gum stimulate and increase saliva, by osmotically drawing water from the tissues, improving pH, and buffering capacity of the saliva in the oral cavity.[40,41] Xylitol is a nonfermentable carbohydrate and inhibits the metabolism of bacterial species, especially mutans streptococci. Xylitol-containing agents aid with the clearance of carbohydrate substrate, dead tissue, and microorganisms, thus reducing the rate of demineralization and inducing remineralization[42] of the hard tissue. This process helps maintain homeostasis of the soft tissue. Recent studies with xylitol lozenges showed a 10% reduction in caries in high risk populations.[43]

SUPERSATURATED CALCIUM AND PHOSPHATE

The use of remineralizing solutions in concentrated doses (eg, Caphosol, Jazz Pharmaceuticals PLC, Dublin, Ireland or Neutrasal, Invado Pharmaceuticals, Pomona, NY, USA) can help provide the physiologic supersaturated level of calcium phosphate that is necessary for remineralization and mucosal healing. This situation is especially so when used with 1.1% Na F amorphous calcium phosphate containing paste, and fortified with 900 ppm fluoride (eg MI Paste and MI Paste Plus, GC America Inc, Alsip, IL, USA). This process may enhance remineralization and decrease demineralization of the calcified tissue in oral cavity.[44,45]

FLUORIDE

Various salts of fluoride are bactericidal and help with the reuptake of calcium and phosphate from the supersaturated saliva and the formation of fluoroapatite crystals, which are more resistant to acidic attacks. Prescription-strength fluoride in the form of toothpastes, gels, and professionally applied varnishes is necessary to prevent caries in a population with salivary hypofunction. Various strengths of fluoride are recommended to people at risk for developing dental carious lesions. As part of the evidence-based approach to care, these clinical recommendations should be integrated with the practitioner's professional judgment and the patient's needs and preferences.[46]

SALIVARY SUBSTITUTES

The evidence for caries protection from salivary substitutes is not sufficient for artificial saliva substitutes. The soothing effect of these substitutes is only temporary and must be administered frequently. Mouth rinses intended to treat dry mouth are expectorated and cleared by swallowing, resulting in only a small residual amount of active agent in the oral cavity. Sprays and gels are also susceptible to rapid dilution as a result of swallowing. Thus, the use of mouth rinses, sprays, and gels is inconvenient and often interruptive of daily activities. The evidence for caries protection is not there for saliva. The Cochrane review reported that,[39] there was no strong evidence for any topical therapy to relieve xerostomia. Oxygenated glycerol triester saliva substitute spray have shown about a 20% improvement over an electrolyte spray.

Commercially available products generally contain mucoadhesive polymers (eg, carboxymethylcellulose or hydroxyethylcellulose), preservatives (eg, methylparaben or propylparaben) and flavoring agents.

REGULAR DENTAL CARE

The frequency of dental office visits for xerostomic elderly patients should be every 3 months. During these visits, the oral cavity should be examined for any development of new dental carious lesions, soft tissue changes to assess any infection or inflammation, review of oral hygiene products, usage of prescriptions, prophylaxis, and most importantly, compliance to the regimen advised to reduce complications in the oral cavity caused by medications.

ACKNOWLEDGMENTS

We would like to thank K.A. Barbera for her editing services.

REFERENCES

1. US Department of Health and Human Services. Centers for Disease Control and Prevention. Health, United States, 2012. With special feature on emergency care. Available at: http://www.cdc.gov/nchs/data/hus/hus12.pdf#018. Accessed December 16, 2013.
2. US Census Bureau, Population division percent distribution of the projected population by selected age groups and sex for the United States: 2015 to 2060. 2012. Available at: http://www.census.gov/population/projections/data/national/2012/summarytables.html. Accessed January 1, 2014.
3. Klotz U. Pharmacokinetics and drug metabolism in the elderly. Drug Metab Rev 2009;41(2):67–76. http://dx.doi.org/10.1080/03602530902722679.
4. Mangoni AA, Jackson SH. Age-related changes in pharmacokinetics and pharmacodynamics: basic principles and practical applications. Br J Clin Pharmacol 2004;57(1):6–14. http://dx.doi.org/10.1046/j.1365-2125.2003.02007.x.
5. Vered M, Buchner A, Boldon P, et al. Age-related histomorphometric changes in labial salivary glands with special reference to the acinar component. Exp Gerontol 2000;35(8):1075–84.
6. Baum BJ. Evaluation of stimulated parotid saliva flow rate in different age groups. J Dent Res 1981;60:1292–6.
7. Nagler RM, Hershkovich O. Age-related changes in unstimulated salivary function and composition and its relations to medications and oral sensorial complaints. Aging Clin Exp Res 2005;17(5):358–66.
8. Centers for Disease Control and Prevention. Prescription drug use continues to increase: US prescription drug data for 2007-2008. Available at: http://www.cdc.gov/nchs/data/databriefs/db42.htm. Accessed January 1, 2014.
9. Farley D. Label literacy for OTC drugs. FDA Consum 1997;31(4):6–11.
10. Glaser J, Rolita L. Educating the older adult in over-the-counter medication use. Geriatr Aging 2009;12(2):103–9.
11. Qato DM, Alexander G, Conti RM, et al. Use of prescription and over-the-counter medications and dietary supplements among older adults in the United States. JAMA 2008;300(24):2867–78. http://dx.doi.org/10.1001/jama.2008.892.
12. Yuan-Pang W, Andrade LH. Epidemiology of alcohol and drug use in the elderly. Curr Opin Psychiatry 2013;26(4):343–8.
13. Feinberg M. The problems of anticholinergic adverse effects of medication in elderly. Arch Intern Med 1993;3:335–48.
14. Mintzer J, Burns A. Anticholinergic side-effects of drugs in elderly people. J R Soc Med 2000;93:457–62.
15. Available at: http://drymouth.info/practitioner/overview.asp. Accessed January 1, 2014.
16. Lambert DG, Appadu BL. Muscarinic receptor subtypes: do they have a place in clinical anesthesia. Br J Anaesth 1995;74:497–9.
17. Available at: https://www.inkling.com/read/pharm-phys-anesthetic-practice-stoelting-4th/chapter-10/ch10-section-2. Accessed January 1, 2014.
18. Tune LE. Anticholinergic effects of medication in elderly patients. J Clin Psychiatry 2001;62(Suppl 21):11–4.
19. Hanlon JT, Schmader KE, Koronkowski MJ, et al. Adverse drug events in high risk older outpatients. J Am Geriatr Soc 1997;45(8):945–8.
20. AGS Beers criteria for potentially inappropriate medication use in older adults. Available at: http://www.americangeriatrics.org/files/documents/beers/Printable BeersPocketCard.pdf. Accessed January 1, 2014.

21. Navazesh M, Christensen C, Brightman V. Clinical criteria for the diagnosis of salivary gland hypofunction. J Dent Res 1992;71(7):1363–9.
22. Sreebny L. Saliva–salivary gland hypofunction (SGH). FDI Working Group 10. J Dent Assoc S Afr 1992;47(11):498–501.
23. Amerongen AV, Veerman EC. Saliva–the defender of the oral cavity. Oral Dis 2002;8:12–22.
24. Vissink A, Spijkervet FK, Van Nieuw Amerongen A. Aging and saliva: a review of the literature. Spec Care Dentist 1996;16(3):95–103.
25. Available at: http://www.umaryland.edu/medmanagement/anticholinergic. Accessed July 28, 2014.
26. Fox PC. Dry mouth: managing the symptoms and providing effective relief. J Clin Dent 2006;17(2):27–9.
27. Turner MD, Ship JA. Dry mouth and its effects on the oral health of elderly people. J Am Dent Assoc 2007;138(Suppl):15S–20S.
28. Sreebny LM, Schwartz SS. A reference guide to drugs and dry mouth–2nd edition. Gerodontology 1997;14:33–47.
29. Featherstone JD. Dental caries: a dynamic disease process. Aust Dent J 2008; 53(3):286–91.
30. Slavkin HC. Maturity and oral health: live longer and better. J Am Dent Assoc 2000;131(6):805–8.
31. Charone S, Portela M, das Chagas M, et al. Biofilm of Candida albicans from oral cavity of an HIV-infected child: challenge on enamel microhardness. Oral Surg Oral Med Oral Pathol Oral Radiol 2013;115(4):500–4. http://dx.doi.org/10.1016/j.oooo.2012.11.003.
32. Signoretto C, Burlacchini G, Faccioni F, et al. Support for the role of Candida spp. in extensive caries lesions of children. New Microbiol 2009; 32(1):101–7.
33. Singh ML, Kugel G, Papas A, et al. Non-carious lesions due to tooth surface loss: to restore or not to restore? Available at: http://cdeworld.com/courses/4496. Inside Dentistry. 2011. Accessed July 28, 2014.
34. Tabak LA, Levine MJ, Mandel ID, et al. Role of salivary mucins in the protection of the oral cavity. J Oral Pathol 1982;11(1):1–17.
35. Moreira TS, Takakura AC, Colombari E, et al. Central moxonidine on salivary gland blood flow and cardiovascular responses to pilocarpine. Brain Res 2003; 987:155–63.
36. Kondo Y, Nakamoto T, Mukaibo T, et al. Cevimeline induced monophasic salivation from the mouse submandibular gland: decreased Na+ content in saliva results from specific and early activation of Na+/H+ Exchange. J Pharmacol Exp Ther 2011;337:267–74.
37. Ono K, Inagaki T, Iida T, et al. Distinct effects of cevimeline and pilocarpine on salivary mechanisms, cardiovascular response and thirst sensation in rats. Arch Oral Biol 2012;57(4):421–8. http://dx.doi.org/10.1016/j.archoralbio.2011.09.013.
38. Dodds MW, Hsieh SC, Johnson DA. The effect of increased mastication by daily gum-chewing on salivary gland output and dental plaque acidogenicity. J Dent Res 1991;70(12):1474–8.
39. Furness S, Worthington HV, Bryan G, et al. Interventions for the management of dry mouth: topical therapies. Cochrane Database Syst Rev 2011;(12):CD008934. http://dx.doi.org/10.1002/14651858.CD008934.pub2.
40. Ribelles Llop M, Guinot Jimeno F, Mayné Acién R, et al. Effects of xylitol chewing gum on salivary flow rate, pH, buffering capacity and presence of Streptococcus mutans in saliva. Eur J Paediatr Dent 2010;11(1):9–14.

41. Aguirre-Zero O, Zero DT, Proskin HM. Effect of chewing xylitol chewing gum on salivary flow rate and the acidogenic potential of dental plaque. Caries Res 1993;27:55–9.
42. Miake Y, Saeki Y, Takahashi M, et al. Remineralization effects of xylitol on demineralized enamel. J Electron Microsc (Tokyo) 2003;52(5):471–6.
43. Bader JD, Vollmer WM, Shugars DA, et al. Results from the Xylitol Adult Caries Trial (X-ACT). J Am Dent Assoc 2013;144(1):21–30.
44. Johansen E, Papas A, Fong W, et al. Remineralization of carious lesions in elderly patients. Gerodontics 1987;3(1):47–50.
45. Singh ML, Papas AS. Long-term clinical observation of dental caries in salivary hypofunction patients using a supersaturated calcium-phosphate remineralizing rinse. J Clin Dent 2009;20(3):87–92.
46. Weyant RJ, Tracy SL, Anselmo TT, et al. Topical fluoride for caries prevention: executive summary of the updated clinical recommendations and supporting systematic review. J Am Dent Assoc 2013;144(11):1279–91.

Systemic Diseases and Oral Health

 CrossMark

Mary Tavares, DMD, MPH[a,b,]*, Kari A. Lindefjeld Calabi, DMD[c],
Laura San Martin, DDS, PhD, MDPH[d]

KEYWORDS

- Chronic illnesses • Diabetes mellitus • Cardiovascular diseases
- Systemic complications

KEY POINTS

- Oral disease management is more complex in patients with several systemic diseases.
- Severe periodontitis adversely affects diabetes control.
- Additional considerations exist for diabetic patients in a dental office setting.
- Osteoarthritis of the hands reduces manual dexterity and constrains the patient's capability of maintaining adequate oral hygiene.

INTRODUCTION

Several new studies have shown that an association exists between oral diseases and systemic chronic diseases. Inflammation has additionally been recognized as the key factor that connects many of these diseases.[1] Chronic diseases are defined as long-lasting illnesses, with duration of more than 3 months that affect a person's life and require constant medical treatment. Chronic diseases more frequently affect aging individuals; 80% have one chronic condition, and 50% have at least 2 conditions.[2] Chronic conditions are the leading cause of death and disability in the United States. According to the National Vital Statistics, the 10 leading causes of death among the 65-years-and-over age group are heart diseases, malignant neoplasm, chronic lower respiratory diseases, cerebrovascular diseases, Alzheimer diseases, diabetes mellitus (DM), influenza and pneumonia, nephritis, unintentional accidents, and septicemia.[3] The authors have chosen to select cardiovascular diseases (CADs), hypertension,

[a] Dental Public Health, Oral Health Policy and Epidemiology, Harvard School of Dental Medicine, 188 Longwood Avenue, Boston, MA 02115, USA; [b] Department of Applied Oral Sciences, The Forsyth Institute, 245 First Street, Cambridge, MA 02142, USA; [c] Oral Health Policy and Epidemiology, Harvard School of Dental Medicine, 188 Longwood Avenue, Boston, MA 02115, USA; [d] Department of Stomatology, School of Dentistry, University of Seville, Avicena, Seville 41009, Spain
* Corresponding author. Dental Public Health, Oral Health Policy and Epidemiology, Harvard School of Dental Medicine, 188 Longwood Avenue, Boston, MA 02115.
E-mail address: mary_tavares@hsdm.harvard.edu

Dent Clin N Am 58 (2014) 797–814
http://dx.doi.org/10.1016/j.cden.2014.07.005
0011-8532/14/$ – see front matter © 2014 Elsevier Inc. All rights reserved.

diabetes, arthritis, osteoporosis, and stroke to discuss in this article. Their connection to oral health is highlighted and oral recommendations are provided. Aspiration pneumonia and cognitive impairment of older adults are discussed in the articles written by Drs Scannapieco, Shay, Brennan, and Strauss.

Fig. 1 shows the percentage of elder individuals affected by one or more chronic diseases.

The complexity of dental treatment in the elderly is greater because of the effects of these chronic diseases, the medications prescribed, and their adverse effects. Systemic diseases can influence oral health, and oral health has an impact on overall health. Social interactions, self-esteem, dietary choices, and nutrition are enhanced by good oral health.

It is important for oral health professionals to understand and recognize the impact of systemic diseases on oral health. With this expanded knowledge, they will be better able to recommend adequate prevention mechanisms and design appropriate oral health treatment plans.

DM

DM is a group of diseases characterized by high levels of blood glucose resulting from defects in insulin production, insulin action, or both. There are 2 main types of diabetes.

- Type 1 diabetes, or insulin-dependent diabetes mellitus (IDDM), is an autoimmune disease that causes the destruction of the insulin-producing β-cells in the pancreas.[4] IDDM is primarily seen in children and younger adults and accounts for approximately 5% of diabetes cases.
- Type 2 diabetes, or noninsulin-dependent diabetes mellitus (NIDDM), is characterized by resistance to insulin and inadequate production of insulin.[5] NIDDM is the most common form of diabetes seen in adults, accounting for between 90% and 95% of cases.

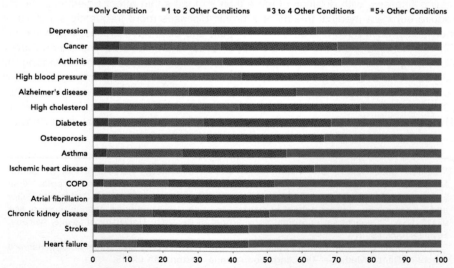

Fig. 1. Co-morbidity among chronic conditions for Medicare fee-for-service beneficiaries, 2010. (*From* Centers for Medicare and Medicaid Services. Chronic conditions among Medicare beneficiaries. Available at: http://www.cms.gov/Research-Statistics-Data-and-Systems/Statistics-Trends-and-Reports/Chronic-Conditions/Downloads/2012Chartbook.pdf. Accessed June 13, 2014.)

- Other types of diabetes including gestational and other genetically specific forms of diabetes account for less than 5% of total diabetes cases.[6]

The following criteria from the American Diabetes Association may be used for the diagnosis of diabetes[7]:

- A1C ≥6.5%. The test is performed in a laboratory using the method of the national glycohemoglobin standardization program certified and standardized to the diabetes control and complication trials assay.
- Fasting plasma glucose ≥126 mg/dL (7.0 mmol/L). Fasting is defined as no caloric intake for at least 8 hours.
- Two-hour plasma glucose ≥200 mg/dL (11.1 mmol/L) during an oral glucose tolerance test using a glucose load containing the equivalent of 75 g anhydrous glucose dissolved in water.
- In a patient with classic symptoms of hyperglycemia or hyperglycemic crisis, a random plasma glucose ≥200 mg/dL (11.1 mmol/L).

Data from the 2011 National Diabetes Fact Sheet show that the prevalence of diabetes in people aged 65 years or older was approximately 26.9% (10.9 million).[6] After adjusting for age and gender, the annual per capita health care expenditure is 2.3 times higher for diabetics than for those without diabetes. Diabetes is especially costly when it presents with complications.[8] It is the seventh leading cause of death in the United States.[6] According to the HealthPartners Dental Group, patients with poorly controlled or uncontrolled diabetes are more susceptible to other illnesses, including periodontal disease.[9,10] Diabetics aged 60 years and older are more likely to be unable to walk one-quarter of a mile or climb stairs when compared with nondiabetics of the same age.[6]

Systemic Complications of Diabetes

- *Heart disease and stroke.* In 2004, heart disease was noted on 68% of diabetes-related death certificates and stroke was noted on 16%. Diabetics have 2 to 4 times greater incidence of stroke and/or heart disease death rates compared with adults without diabetes.[6]
- *Hypertension and dyslipidemia* are risk factors for CVD, and diabetes itself confers an independent risk.[11]
- *Blindness and ocular problems.* The leading cause of new cases of blindness among adults is diabetes.[6]
- *Kidney disease.* Diabetes is the leading cause of kidney failure, accounting for 44% of all new cases of kidney failure in 2008.[6]
- *Neurologic problems.* About 60% to 70% of people with diabetes suffer from some degree of nerve damage including impaired sensation on feet or hands, slowed digestion of food in the stomach, or other neurologic problems.[6]
- *Amputations.* Peripheral neuropathy and decreased pain sensation has been shown to increase the risk of skin breakdown and severe nonhealing infections. More than 60% of nontraumatic lower-limb amputations occur in people with diabetes.
- *Mental health.* People with diabetes have twice the risk of depression. Depression is also associated with a 60% increase of developing type 2 diabetes. Diabetes management is further complicated by mental illness because it often leads to poor patient compliance. Patients with diabetes may also experience anxiety, stress, and anger.[6,12]
- *Hearing loss.* According to the American Diabetes Association, hearing loss is twice as common in people with diabetes. The results of a 2013 study revealed

a close link between audiovestibular dysfunction and diabetes. Based on these findings, vestibular dysfunction and sensorineural hearing loss may be considered among the chronic complications due to NIDDM.[13]

Oral Health Implications of Diabetes

- *Gingivitis and periodontal disease.* Periodontitis is the major cause of tooth loss in elderly subjects and is considered to be the sixth complication of DM.[14,15] Adults aged 45 years and older with poorly controlled diabetes (A1C >9%) are 2.9 times more likely to have severe periodontitis than those without diabetes. The likelihood is even greater (4.6 times) among smokers with poorly controlled diabetes.[6] Diabetes also delays healing and increases the risk of oral infection and abscess formation.

A recent Korean study of an elderly population demonstrated the relationship between metabolic conditions and the prevalence of periodontal disease. The results showed that participants with longer durations of diabetes, high blood pressure, and obesity were significantly more likely to have periodontal disease.[16]

Periodontal disease is associated with hyperglycemia and poor control of diabetes. The association is considered to be bidirectional: diabetes is a risk of periodontitis and periodontitis is a possible severity factor for diabetes.[17]

Diabetes induces the formation of AGE (advanced glycation end-products), elevates cytokines levels, and enhances oxidative stress in periodontal tissues exacerbating periodontal disease. However, periodontal treatment can play an important role in controlling diabetes by reducing plasma HbA1C at 3 months by levels equivalent to adding a second drug to a pharmacologic regimen (**Fig. 2**).[18]

- *Xerostomia* is dryness of the mouth, which is caused by salivary dysfunction. Researchers in Macedonia concluded that there is a significant correlation between the degree of xerostomia and salivary levels of glucose.[19] Salivary

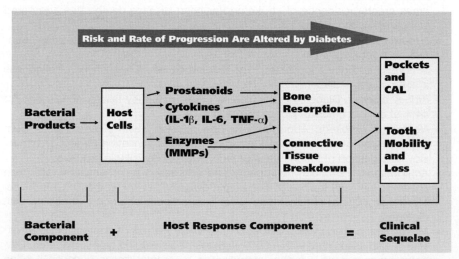

Fig. 2. Simplified schematic depicting etiologic factors and cascade of events contributing to periodontitis that are altered by diabetes. CAL, clinical attachment loss; IL-1β, interleukin-1β; IL-6, interleukin-6; MMPs, matrix metalloproteinases; TNF-α, tumor necrosis factor-α. (*From* Ryan ME, Carnu O, Kamer A. The influence of diabetes on the periodontal tissues. J Am Dent Assoc 2003;134:34S–40S; with permission.)

hypofunction leads to dry and friable oral mucosa, decrease in lubrication, decreased antimicrobial activity, increased caries activity, increased oral fungal infections, glossodynia, dysgeusia, dysphagia, difficulty with mastication, and impaired retention of removable prostheses.[20] Elderly populations are more often affected by xerostomia because of a higher prevalence of systemic diseases and the increased use of prescription drugs.

- *Dental caries* have been found to be more common and more severe in diabetic patients. A decreased salivary flow rate, along with poor glycemic control and significantly increased value of HbA1C, was found to be associated with a higher number of carious teeth. Further research is needed to establish a better role for salivary flow rate and minerals with regard to dental caries of diabetic patients.[21]
- *Oral mucosa lesions.* Studies have shown that specific lesions, such as geographic tongue, denture stomatitis, and angular cheilitis, occur with significantly greater frequency among diabetics.[22,23] The cause of geographic tongue in diabetics is still unknown, but may be associated with slower repair and delayed healing caused by the microangiopathy of the oral vasculature in diabetic patients.[22]
- *Fungal infections.* Several researchers have reported that diabetics have an increased predisposition to oral candidiasis, denture stomatitis, and angular cheilitis.[24] There is a high incidence of candidiasis as well as a secondary relationship with salivary dysfunction in diabetic patients.

Drug Interactions and Effects

Polypharmacy is a constant issue in the care of geriatric patients. For this reason, potential interactions with medications should always be considered when administering or prescribing any drugs in the dental setting.

- Insulin, a hormone used to treat IDDM, is compatible with most medications prescribed in the dental office. However, extended doses of aspirin can enhance the hypoglycemic effect of insulin.[25] Consequently, these drugs should not be used for prolonged periods of time.
- Metformin is an oral antidiabetic drug that may cause an increased hypoglycemic effect with extended use of nonsteroidal anti-inflammatory drugs (NSAIDs) and aspirin. Similarly, the tablet form of the antifungal agent Ketoconazole can also enhance this hypoglycemic effect.[26] Long-term use of metformin can lead to vitamin B12 deficiency.[27] This deficiency is associated with atrophic glossitis, angular cheilitis, candidiasis, and recurrent aphthous stomatitis.[28]
- The quantity of epinephrine contained in the dental anesthetic has no significant effect on the diabetic patient's blood sugar level.[29]

Recommendations for Providing Dental Care to Diabetics

- Dental providers should assess glycemic control routinely before any invasive procedures.
- Patients should be asked about any changes in insulin dosage, hypoglycemic medications, and diet before their dental appointment.
- Consultations with an interdisciplinary health team should be done when needed.
- Routine screening for diabetes complications and close monitoring of patients should be done at each visit.
- The oral health provider should emphasize preventive procedures, periodic oral examinations, and prevention of periodontal disease. Patients with diabetes require good oral hygiene habits for maintenance of their oral health.

HYPERTENSION

Hypertension is defined as systolic blood pressure greater than 140 mm Hg or diastolic blood pressure greater than 90 mm Hg. It is one of the most common and potentially dangerous medical conditions among the elderly, affecting approximately two-thirds of men and three-quarters of women 75 years and older.[30,31]

The World Health Organization (WHO) describes hypertension as a global public health issue. In the United States, about 77.9 million (1 of every 3) adults have high blood pressure, and future projections suggest that the prevalence will increase by 7.2% by 2030 (**Table 1**).[32]

It is very important to routinely measure blood pressure at each geriatric patient's dental appointment. Hypertension is called "the silent killer" because individuals do not present with signs or symptoms and may not realize they have it. Hypertension presents differently in elderly and younger people. **Box 1** summarizes the specific features of hypertension among the elderly.[30]

Systemic Complications of Hypertension

- Hypertension is associated with shorter overall life expectancy and a shorter life free of CVD.
- Atherosclerosis is caused when hypertension damages the endothelium in the wall of the blood vessels[33]; it affects the aorta and its major branches, the coronary artery and the larger cerebral artery. The arterial changes include the narrowing of the lumen of the vessels, weakening of the arterioles, and eventual rupture of the vessel. Atherosclerosis is a common cause of myocardial infarctions and cerebrovascular accidents.[34]
- CVDs are associated with advanced hypertension. About 50% of people who suffer a first heart attack have blood pressure greater than 160/95 mm Hg.[35] Reducing diastolic blood pressure from 90 mm Hg to 80 mm Hg in a study of people with diabetes reduced the risk of major cardiovascular events by 50%.[36]
- Cerebrovascular accident or stroke constitutes the leading cause of death in the United States and is also the leading cause of serious long-term disability. High blood pressure, high low-density lipoprotein cholesterol, and smoking are the key risk factors for strokes.[37] Approximately 66% of people experiencing a first stroke have high blood pressure.[35]
- Increased blood pressure can cause dilation of the wall of an artery or vein, forming an aneurysm. If an aneurysm ruptures, it can be life-threatening.
- Hypertensive retinopathy refers to the rupture and hemorrhage of the retinal arterioles. Examination of the eyes may show early changes of hypertension consisting of narrowed arterioles with sclerosis.
- Alzheimer disease and hypertension are major determinants of cognitive dysfunction and are associated with alterations in the structure and function of

Table 1
Hypertension among elder adult populations (2007–2010)

	65–74 y	75 + y
Men	64.1%	71.7%
Women	69.3%	81.3%

Data from National Center for Health Statistics. Health, United States, 2012: Table 64. Hypertension among adults aged 20 and over, by selected characteristics: United States, selected years 1988–1994 through 2009–2012. Hyattsville (MD): 2013. Available at: http://www.cdc.gov/nchs/data/hus/2012/064.pdf. Accessed August 1, 2014.

> **Box 1**
> **Features of hypertension among the elderly**
>
> - Elevated systolic blood pressure (BP) is more common in the elderly
> - Impaired baroreflex sensitivity (receptor responsible to buffer blood pressure against sudden changes in posture)
> - Variability in blood pressure during daily activities
> - Hypotension during activities such as standing upright and eating
> - Association with cognitive and functional decline
> - CVD or sleep apnea increases BP at night or awakening
>
> *Adapted from* Lipsitz LA. A 91-year-old woman with difficult-to-control hypertension: a clinical review. JAMA 2013;310(12):1274–80.

cerebral vessels. These vascular alterations may impair delivery of energy substrates and nutrients to the brain and impede the clearance of potentially toxic products.[38] A systematic review published in September 2013 showed the paucity of research addressing the association between hypertension and dementia. The available data point toward antihypertensives being effective in lowering blood pressure in people with mild to moderate dementia, but there is no evidence of benefit in cognitive outcomes.[39]

- Hypertensive nephropathy or end-stage renal disease is closely related to chronic hypertension.

Oral Health Implications of Hypertension

- Drugs used for the treatment of hypertension can cause xerostomia, which potentially causes extensive tooth decay, mouth sores, and oral infections. Patients with xerostomia often complain of difficulty in swallowing and glossodynia. Thiazide diuretics, α-/β-blockers, angiotensin-converting-enzymes inhibitors, and calcium channel blockers increase the risk of xerostomia.[40]
- The Puerto Rican Elderly Dental Health Study suggests that periodontitis may contribute to poor blood pressure control among adults.[41] However, more studies are needed to ascertain this finding.
- Gingival hyperplasia is a side effect of Nifedipine, Diltiazepan, Verapamil, and Amlodipine (calcium channel blockers) used in the treatment of hypertension.[42] In severe cases, surgical removal of tissue may be required.[43]
- Mucosa lesions such as lichenoid reactions may also be caused by several hypertensive medications.

Drug Interactions and Effects

- Diuretics are the drugs mostly used for the management of hypertension. NSAIDs can decrease the efficacy of thiazide diuretics and β-blockers if used for more than 5 days.[44,45] Elderly patients should be prescribed the lowest effective NSAID dose for the shortest duration possible. NSAIDs may also induce new onset hypertension or worsen pre-existing hypertension. Blood pressure should be routinely monitored in patients prescribed NSAIDs.[46]
- Patients medicated with nonselective β-blockers are at risk for acute hypertensive episodes if they receive vasopressors (ie, epinephrine) in local anesthetics.[45] α-/β-Blockers and diuretics may potentiate the actions of anti-anxiety medications and sedative drugs.[47]

- β-Blockers affect the central nervous system and may cause orthostatic hypotension resulting in fainting and falls after a patient gets up from the dental chair.[48] The prevalence of orthostatic hypotension is higher in older community-dwelling adults with uncontrolled hypertension than in those with controlled hypertension.[49]
- Calcium blockers cause vasodilation and reduction in heart rate.[50]
- Calcium blockers, such as Verapamil and Diltiazem, compete with macrolide antibiotics, such as erythromycin and azithromycin, for liver metabolism. The potentially elevated levels of macrolides could result in cardiac toxicity, and elevated levels of calcium blockers can cause bradycardias and atrioventricular block.[50]

Recommendations for Providing Dental Care to Hypertensive Patients

- Measure a patient's blood pressure before the initiation of any dental treatment. Follow guidelines noted in **Box 1**.
- Consultation with an interdisciplinary team may be needed to establish a parameter in which a patient can be safely treated in the dental office.
- Use caution when administrating local anesthetics that contain epinephrine. Limit their usage to 1 or 2 cartridges of 2% lidocaine with 1:100,000 epinephrine.
- In patients with uncontrolled and severe hypertension, anesthetics without vasoconstrictors should be used. Vasoconstrictors impregnated in gingival cords should also be avoided.
- Minimize the potential of orthostatic hypotension by raising the dental chair gradually and allowing the patient to remain in an upright seated position before standing.[49]
- Reduce stress and anxiety to avoid an acute elevation in blood pressure as a result of the released of endogenous catecholamines (**Table 2**).

CVDs

CVD refers to any disease that affects the heart, the blood vessels (arteries, capillaries, and veins), or both. The causes of CVD are diverse. Some risk factors can be controlled through lifestyle changes and/or medications, such as hypertension, hypercholesterolemia, obesity, diabetes, unhealthy diet, stress, tobacco use, and physical inactivity. On the other hand, nonmodifiable risk factors include advanced age, inherited disposition, gender, and ethnicity.

Table 2
Dental management and follow-up recommendations based on blood pressure levels

Blood Pressure	Dental Treatment	Referral to Physician
≤120/80	Any required	No
≥120/80 but <140/90	Any required	Encourage patient to see physician
≥140/90 but <160/100	Any required	Encourage patient to see physician
≥169/100 but <180/110	Any required; continuous monitoring of blood pressure during procedure	Refer patient to physician within 1 mo
≥180/110	Defer elective treatment	Refer patient as soon as possible; if patient is symptomatic, refer immediately

From Little JW, Falace DA, Miller CS, et al. Little and Falace's dental management of the medically compromised patient. 8th edition. Philadelphia: Elsevier; 2012; with permission.

The preferred clinical approach to cardiovascular prevention is to address all modifiable risk factors and support healthier lifestyles in the community. A healthy diet, moderate physical activity, and smoking cessation can prevent 80% of premature heart disease.[51] Heart disease is the leading cause of death in the United States, accounting for 1 in every 4 deaths.[52]

CVDs include:

- Coronary heart disease is the most common type of heart disease, occurring when the coronary arteries become narrowed or blocked as a result of the formation of plaques within the artery walls, reducing blood flow to the heart.
- Peripheral artery disease refers to the obstruction of large arteries (outside the heart and brain) from atherosclerosis. As a result of the inflammatory process, stenosis, thrombus, or embolism can develop.
- Cerebrovascular disease refers to a group of dysfunctions that affect the circulation of blood to the brain. Ischemic or hemorrhagic events result in tissue necrosis and neuronal injury (stroke). Stroke remains one of the major public health problems in the United States; approximately 795,000 new or recurrent cases occur each year.[53]

Oral Health Complications of CVDs

No oral manifestations are related to CVDs per se; however, side effects of medications used to treat CVDs affect the oral cavity. Dry mouth, burning of the mouth, taste changes, and lichenoid reactions are linked to side effects of heart failure medications.[54]

Epidemiologic evidence suggests an association among periodontal infections, atherosclerosis, and vascular disease. According to the American Academy of Periodontology, periodontal disease may double the likelihood of having coronary artery disease. The relationship between CVD and periodontal disease may be explained by different biological mechanisms.[55]

Dental professionals should follow the American Heart Association guidelines for antibiotic prophylaxis for those patients at risk of bacterial endocarditis.[56] Some patients on long-term anticoagulant therapy (Coumadin) are at an increased risk of excessive bleeding during surgical procedures. Dentists should consult with their patients' physicians about the type of procedure and the level of the international normalized ratio (INR). For patients who have stable INR, in the therapeutic range 2 to 4, oral anticoagulants should not be discontinued, even in cases where the patient requires a dental extraction.[57]

Patients on antiplatelet therapy, such as aspirin combined with clopidogrel/dipyridamole, could have increased postoperative bleeding after dental procedures. However, this bleeding can be managed using local haemostatic measures.

Drug Interactions and Effects

Digitalis glycosides is used to increase the myocardial contractility in patients with congestive heart failure. If digoxin toxicity occurs, signs and symptoms include hypersalivation, nausea, and vomiting. Digoxin may also increase the gag reflex.[58]

Because hypertension is a risk factor for stroke, many stroke patients take antihypertensive medications, such as β-blockers, calcium channel blockers, and anti-arrhythmics. Therefore, the same considerations as described in the section of hypertensive patients should be taken into account.

Recommendations for Providing Dental Care to Patients with CVDs

- Evaluate vital signs before any dental procedure.
- Schedule short appointments, preferably in the morning.
- Use caution when administering epinephrine (maximum 0.036 mg epinephrine or 0.20 mg levonordefrin) and anticholinergics; the use of these drugs may lead to cardiac excitation.[58]
- For patients taking digoxin, avoid the use of vasoconstrictors; these may cause arrhythmias. Watch for signs of digoxin toxicity, such as hypersalivation, because macrolide and tetracycline antibiotics may lead to digoxin toxicity.[58]
- Avoid the use of NSAIDs.[58]
- Avoid the use of gingival retraction cords impregnated with epinephrine in all patients with CVDs. Use alternatives such as tetrahydrozoline HCl 0.05% or ocymetazoline HCl 0.05%.
- Be cautious when using electrical devices that might interfere (eg, ultrasound scalers) in patients with pacemakers or implantable defibrillators.[59]
- The INR or the prothrombin time laboratory values should be measured when performing dental procedures in patients with anticoagulant therapy to assure that they are in the acceptable range.

CEREBROVASCULAR DISEASE

Stroke is a cerebrovascular disorder characterized by a sudden interruption of blood flow to the brain, causing oxygen deprivation. It is frequently seen in patients with current CVDs.[60] Stroke is the fourth leading cause of death in the United States and a major cause of adult disability.[32,61]

Systemic Complications of Stroke

- Cardiac complications, such as myocardial infarction, cardiac arrhythmias, congestive heart failure, and cardiomyopathy, can occur after a stroke.[62]
- Pulmonary complications, such as pneumonia, are the most frequent complications within the first 48 hours after a stroke. Most stroke-related pneumonias result from aspiration.[63]
- Gastrointestinal complications, such as dysphagia, which could lead to restriction of oral intake, can cause malnutrition and dehydration in stroke patients.[64]
- Genitourinary complications, including urinary incontinence and urinary tract infections, delay hospital discharge and can lead to institutionalization of patients.[65]
- Venous thromboembolism, some of which are deep vein thrombosis and pulmonary embolism, can occur within 2 weeks after a stroke.[62]
- Other complications include depression, pain, fatigue, decubitus ulcers, hip fractures, immobility, or being bedridden.

Oral Health Complications of Stroke

Stroke patients are very vulnerable to oral diseases because of the limitations in the activities of daily living and impaired manual dexterity.[66] Inadequate oral hygiene combined with xerostomia leads to additional oral problems, such as candidiasis, dental caries, periodontitis, mucosal lesions, and tooth loss.

Drug Interactions and Effects

These drug interactions and effects are similar to those discussed in the CVDs section.

Recommendations for Providing Dental Care to Patients Affected by Stroke

- More frequent recall appointments are recommended and preventive oral care is critical.
- Electric toothbrush or adaptive holders are recommended when impaired manual dexterity exists.
- Dentists should defer elective and invasive dental care for patients within the first 3 months after a stroke.
- Seat the patient in an upright position and use caution to avoid aspiration of foreign objects by the patient during dental treatment.[67]

ARTHRITIS

Arthritis is a musculoskeletal disorder characterized by the inflammation of one or more joints, causing pain and stiffness in the affected joints.[68] There are more than 100 types of arthritis; some of the more common types include osteoarthritis (OA), rheumatoid arthritis, systemic lupus erythematosus, Lyme disease, scleroderma, gout, fibromyalgia, and psoriadic arthritis.[69]

OA is a degenerative joint disease that is the most common form of arthritis among the elderly. OA affects both men and woman, but after age 45, it is more common in women.[70] An estimated 27 million adults had OA in 2005, and 50% of those 65 and older were diagnosed with the condition.[71,72] OA is the most common form of joint disease and is a leading cause of disability in elderly people.[73]

There is no cure for arthritis; treatments serve to reduce pain, improve function, and slow disease progression. Acetaminophen is recommended as a first-line drug, with aspirin and NSAIDs also commonly used. Narcotic analgesics and intra-articular steroid injections are reserved for acute flares over short periods of time. Surgery, including joint replacement, may be indicated to improve function.[47]

Oral Health Implications of Arthritis

- Arthritis can affect the temporomandibular joint, compromising the range of jaw aperture and affecting mastication.
- OA of the hands causes pain and reduces manual dexterity, which can affect oral hygiene by making routine brushing and flossing more challenging.
- Patients with prosthetic joints need antibiotic prophylaxis before invasive dental treatment to prevent oral bacteria from traveling through the bloodstream to the prosthetic joint. Dental providers should follow the updated guidelines by the American Academy of Orthopaedic Surgeons for antibiotic prophylaxis for patients with joint replacements.

Drug Interactions and Effects

- Aspirin and NSAIDs may increase bleeding during dental procedures, but it is usually not clinically significant.[69,74,75]
- As previously noted, blood pressure should be routinely monitored in patients taking NSAIDs because these drugs may induce new onset hypertension or worsen pre-existing hypertension by causing fluid retention or edema.[46]

Recommendations for Providing Dental Care to Patients with Arthritis

- The use of an electric toothbrush and floss with a long handle can facilitate daily oral hygiene for patients with manual limitations.
- Short appointments are preferable in patients with multiple joint problems because these patients may have joint discomfort and pain in numerous regions

of their bodies. Patients should also be allowed to adjust their positioning as needed.[69]

- Additional pillows, cushioning, and/or adjustments of the dental chair can aid in patient comfort.
- For patients with removable partial dentures, clasps should be designed to maximize ease of placement and removal.

OSTEOPOROSIS

Osteoporosis is defined as a skeletal disorder that compromises bone strength, predisposing a person to an increased risk of bone fracture due to inhibited calcium intake and mineral loss. Osteoporosis can be characterized as either primary or secondary. Primary osteoporosis occurs in both genders at all ages, but typically follows menopause in women and occurs later in life in men. Secondary osteoporosis is the result of medications (glucocorticoids), other conditions (hypogonadism), or diseases (celiac disease, cystic fibrosis).[76]

Osteoporosis has been defined from bone mineral density (BMD) assessment. According to the WHO criteria, osteoporosis is defined as a BMD 2.5 SDs or more less than the average value for young healthy women (a T score of < -2.5 SD).[77]

The National Osteoporosis Foundation estimates that more than 10 million people over the age of 50 have osteoporosis and another 34 million are at risk for the disease. Bone fractures among the elderly reduce mobility and potentially increase the need for long-term care. Hip fractures are particularly problematic; 1 in 3 older adults who lived independently before a hip fracture remained in a nursing home for at least 1 year after their injury.[78]

Oral Health Implications of Osteoporosis

Studies have shown that mandibular and maxillary bone densities, as well as alveolar BMD and height, are modestly correlated with other skeletal sites. However, whether low BMD in the jaw results in other adverse changes, such as missing teeth, gingival bleeding, greater probing depth, and gingival recession, is still unclear.[79]

Drug Interactions and Effects

Bisphosphonates are the primary drugs used to treat osteoporosis by suppressing osteoclast activity and increasing BMD. Intravenous (IV) bisphosphonates are used in the treatment of certain malignancies, skeletal-related events associated with bone metastases, and multiple myeloma. Oral bisphosphonates are used to treat osteoporosis and osteopenia (decrease of calcification and bone density). Patients treated with IV bisphosphonates have a risk of developing bisphosphonates-related osteonecrosis of the jaw (BRONJ). This risk increases when the duration of the therapy exceeds 3 years.[80] Patients taking oral bisphosphonates are at a considerably lower risk.[81]

According to the American Academy of Oral and Maxillofacial Surgeons, patients with BRONJ present all of the following characteristics: current or previous treatment with bisphosphonates, exposed bone in the maxillofacial region that has persisted for more than 8 weeks, and no history of radiation to the jaw.[82,83]

Recommendations for Providing Dental Care to Patients with Osteoporosis

- Dentists should be aware of the implications and possible risks when patients are under bisphosphonates therapy.[84]

Table 3
Dental treatment recommendations for patients treated with bisphosphonates

Patient Therapy with Bisphosphonates	Recommended Oral Treatment
• Oral bisphosphonate therapy • Beginning IV bisphosphonate therapy • IV bisphosphonate therapy for <3 mo with no osteonecrosis of the jaw	• Treat active oral infections • Eliminate sites at high risk for infection • Remove nonrestorable teeth and teeth with substantial periodontal bone loss • Encourage routine dental care, oral examinations, and cleanings. Minimization of periodontal inflammation, restorative treatment of caries, and endodontic therapy where indicated
• IV bisphosphonate therapy for 3 mo or more with no osteonecrosis of the jaw	• Seek alternatives to surgical oral procedures with appropriate local and systemic antibiotics • Conduct extractions and other surgery using as little bone manipulation as possible, appropriate local and systemic antibiotics, and close follow-up to monitor healing
• Bisphosphonate therapy with osteonecrosis of the jaw	• Follow all recommendations for group 2 above • Consider additional imaging studies such as computed tomography scans. • Remove necrotic bone as necessary with minimal trauma to adjacent tissue • Prescribe oral rinses, such as chlorhexidine gluconate 0.12% • Prescribe systemic antibiotics and analgesics if needed • Fabricate a soft acrylic stent to cover areas of exposed bone, protect adjacent soft tissues, and improve comfort[85] • Suggest cessation of bisphosphonate therapy until osteonecrosis heals or the underlying diseases progresses (discussion with patient's medical providers)

Adapted from Kelsey JL. Musculoskeletal conditions. In: Lamster IB, Northridge ME. Improving oral health for the elderly. New York: Springer; 2008; with permission.

- The recommendations to dental professionals for managing patients on bisphosphonates therapy are presented in **Table 3**.

SUMMARY

This article summarizes some of the most common systemic diseases affecting the elderly population. Preventive approaches are emphasized and recommendations are offered for patient management to provide an improved understanding of systemic disease complications affecting the oral and systemic health of older patients.

REFERENCES

1. Freire MO, Van Dyke TE. The oral-systemic health connection. A guide to patient care. In: Glick M, editor. Chapter 5: the mechanisms behind oral-systemic

interactions. 1st edition. Chicago: International Quintessence Publishing Group; 2014. p. 103–17.

2. Available at: http://www.cdc.gov/chronicdisease/resources/publications/aag/pdf/2011/healthy_aging_aag_508.pdf. Accessed November 10, 2013.

3. National Vital Statistics Reports, vol. 62, December 20, 2013. Table 1. Deaths, percentage of total deaths, and death rates for the 10 leading causes of death in selected age groups, by race and sex: United Sates, 2010-Con. Available at: http://www.cdc.gov/nchs/data/nvsr/nvsr62/nvsr62_06.pdf. Accessed November 10, 2013.

4. Marron MP, Raffel LJ, Garchon HJ, et al. Insulin-dependent diabetes mellitus (IDDM) is associated with CTLA4 polymorphisms in multiple ethnic groups. Hum Mol Genet 1997;6(8):1275–82. http://dx.doi.org/10.1093/hmg/6.8.1275.

5. Maitra A. The endocrine system. In: Kumar V, Abbas AK, Fausto N, et al, editors. Robbins basic pathology. 8th edition. Philadelphia: W.B. Saunders Company; 2008. p. 751–76.

6. Centers for Disease Control and Prevention. National diabetes fact sheet: national estimates and general information on diabetes and prediabetes in the United States, 2011. Atlanta (GA): U.S. Department of Health and Human Services, Centers for Disease Control and Prevention; 2011. Available at: http://www.cdc.gov/diabetes/pubs/pdf/ndfs_2011.pdf. Accessed October 9, 2013.

7. Available at: http://care.diabetesjournals.org/content/36/Supplement_1/S11/T2.expansion.htm. Accessed November 11, 2013.

8. American Diabetes Association. Economic Costs of Diabetes in the U.S. in 2012. Diabetes Care 2013;36(4):1033–46.

9. Dental Considerations for Geriatric Patients. CME resource. 2013. p. 12. Available at: http://www.netce.com/839/Course_3956.pdf. Accessed August 1, 2014.

10. Dental Considerations for Geriatric Patients. CME resource. 2013. p. 12. Available at: http://www.netce.com/coursecontent.php?courseid=842. Accessed November 12, 2013.

11. Available at: http://care.diabetesjournals.org/content/36/Supplement_1/S11.full. Accessed November 11, 2013.

12. Available at: http://www.diabetes.org/living-with-diabetes/complications/mental-health/. Accessed November 16, 2013.

13. Özel HE, Özkiris M, Gencer ZK, et al. Audiovestibular functions in noninsulin-dependent diabetes mellitus. Acta Otolaryngol 2014;134:51–7.

14. Wolf DL, Papapanou PN. The relationship and systemic disease in the elderly. In: Lamster IB, Northridge ME, editors. Improving oral health for the elderly. New York: Springer; 2008. p. 247–71.

15. Loe H. Periodontal disease. The sixth complication of diabetes mellitus. Diabetes Care 1993;16(1):329.

16. Lee KS, Kim EK, Kim JW, et al. The relationship between metabolic conditions and prevalence of periodontal disease in rural Korean elderly. Arch Gerontol Geriatr 2014;58(1):125–9.

17. Wolf DL, Papapanou PN. The relationship between periodontal disease and systemic disease in the elderly. Chapter 12. In: Lamster IB, Northridge ME, editors. Improving oral health for the elderly. New York: Springer; 2008. p. 247–71.

18. Chapple IL, Genco R, Working group 2 of the joint EFP/AAP workshop. Diabetes and periodontal diseases:consensus report of the joint EFP/AAP workshop on periodontitis and systemic diseases. J Periodontol 2013;84(4 Suppl):S106–12. http://dx.doi.org/10.1902/jop.2013.1340011.

19. Ivanovski K, Naumovski V, Kostadinova M, et al. Xerostomia and salivary levels of glucose and urea in patients with diabetes. Prilozi 2012;33:219–29. Available at: http://www.manu.edu.mk/prilozi/2012_2/18i.pdf. Accessed November 16, 2013.

20. Ship JA. Oral medicine in geriatrics. In: Clinician's guide. Oral health in geriatric patients. 2nd edition. Hamilton, Ontario: BC Decker Inc; 2006. p. 1–5.

21. Jawed M, Shahid SM, Qader SA, et al. Dental caries in diabetes mellitus: role of salivary flow rate and minerals. J Diabetes Complications 2011;25(3):183–6.

22. Al-Maweri SA, Ismail NM, Ismail AR, et al. Prevalence of oral mucosal lesions in patients with tye 2 diabetes attending Universiti Sains Malaysia. Malays J Med Sci 2013;20(4):39–46.

23. Gandara B, Morton T. Non-Periodontal oral manifestations of diabetes: a framework for medical care providers. Diabetes Spectr 2011;24(4):199–205.

24. Lalla RV, D'Ambrosio JA. Dental management considerations for the patient with diabetes mellitus. J Am Dent Assoc 2001;132:1425–32.

25. Appendix C. Drug interactions of significance to dentistry. Table c-1. In: Little JW, editor. Dental management of the medically compromised patient. 6th edition. Missouri: Mosby; 2002. p. 541–70.

26. Insulin, oral hypoglycemics, and glucagon. Chapter 36. In: Yagiela JA, editor. Pharmacology and therapeutics for dentistry. 5th edition. Missouri: Mosby; 2004. p. 573–82.

27. de Jager J, Kooy A, Lehert P, et al. Long term treatment with metformin in patients with type 2 diabetes and risk of vitamin B-12 deficiency: randomized placebo controlled trial. BMJ 2010;340:c2181. http://dx.doi.org/10.1136/bmj.c2181.

28. Field EA, Speechley JA, Rugman FR, et al. Oral signs and symptoms in patients with undiagnosed vitamin B12 deficiency. J Oral Pathol Med 1995;24(10): 468–70. http://dx.doi.org/10.1111/1600-0714.ep11339775.

29. Box 31.14 Principles of dental management of diabetics. In: Cawson RA, editor. Cawson's essentials of oral pathology and oral medicine e-book. 8th edition. Edinburgh: Churchill Livingstone; 2012. VitalBook file.

30. Lipsitz LA. A 91-year-old woman with difficult-to-control hypertension. A clinical review. JAMA 2013;310:1274–80. Available at: http://jama.jamanetwork.com.ezp-prod1.hul.harvard.edu/article.aspx?articleid=1741837. Accessed November 24, 2013.

31. Lloyd-Jones D, Adams R, Camethon M, et al, American Heart Association Statistics Committee and Stroke Statistics Subcommittee. Heart disease and stroke statistics- 2009 update. Circulation 2009;119(3):e21–181.

32. Go AS, Mozaffarian D, Roger VL, et al. Heart disease and stroke statistics-2013 update: a report from the American Heart Association. Circulation 2013;127: e6–245. http://dx.doi.org/10.1161/CIR.0bo13e31828124ad. Available at: http://www.cdc.gov/Other/disclaimer.html.

33. Chapter 14. Smooth muscle. In: Koeppen BM, editor. Berne & Levy physiology. 6th edition. Philadelphia: Mosby; 2008. p. 268–85.

34. Bots ML, Hoes AW, Koudstaal PJ, et al. Common carotid intima-media thickness and risks of stroke and myocardial infartation. The Rotterdam study. Circulation 1997;96:1432–7. Available at: http://circ.ahajournals.org/content/96/5/1432.short.

35. Magnus P, Beaglehole R. The real contribution of the major risk factors to the coronary epidemics. Arch Intern Med 2001;161:2657–60.

36. Available at: http://www.cdc.gov/diabetes/pubs/pdf/ndfs_2011.pdf. Accessed November 24, 2013.

37. Centers for Disease Control and Prevention. Stroke facts. Available at: http://www.cdc.gov/stroke/facts.htm. Accessed November 24, 2013.

38. Iadecola C, Park L, Capone C. Threats to the mind: aging, amyloid, and hypertension. Stroke 2009;40(3 Suppl):S40–4. http://dx.doi.org/10.1161/STROKEAHA. 108.5336338.

39. Beishon LC, Harrison JK, Harwood RH, et al. The evidence for treating hypertension in older people with dementia: a systematic review. J Hum Hypertens 2014; 28:283–7. Available at: http://www.nature.com.ezp-prod1.hul.harvard.edu/jhh/journal/vaop/ncurrent/pdf/jhh2013107a.pdf.

40. Herman WW, Konzelman JL Jr, Prisant LM, Joint National Committee on Prevention, Detection, Evaluation, and Treatment of High Blood Pressure. New national guidelines on hypertension. A summary for dentistry. J Am Dent Assoc 2004; 135:576–84.

41. Southerland JH. Periodontitis may contribute to poor control of hypertension in older adults. J Evid Based Dent Pract 2013;13(3):125–7.

42. Kerr AR, Phelan JA. Benign lesions of the oral cavity. Chapter 6. Drug-induced gingival enlargement. In: Greenberg MS, editor. Burket's oral medicine. 11th edition. Hamilton: B.C. Decker; 2007. p. 129–52.

43. Dental Considerations for Geriatric Patients. CME resource. 2013. p. 8. Available at: http://www.netce.com/839/Course_3956.pdf. Accessed November 25, 2013.

44. Dental Considerations for Geriatric Patients. CME resource. 2013. p. 7. Available at: http://www.netce.com/839/Course_3956.pdf. Accessed August 1, 2014.

45. Becker DE. Cardiovascular drugs: implications for dental practice part 1- cardiotonics, diuretics and vasodilators. Anesth Prog 2007;54:178–86 DDS2007 by the American Dental Society of Anesthesiology. p. 180. Available at: http://www.ncbi.nlm.nih.gov/pmc/articles/PMC2213250/.

46. Texas Health and Human Services Commission. Criteria for outpatient Use Guidelines. Nonsteroidal Anti-Inflammatory Drugs. Available at: http://www.txvendordrug.com/downloads/criteria/nsaids.shtml. Accessed November 15, 2013.

47. Little JW, Falace DA, Miller CS, et al. Hypertension. In: Dental management of the medically compromised patient. 7th edition. Missouri: Mosby; 2008. p. 34–66.

48. Dental Considerations for Geriatric Patients. CME resource. 2013. p. 6. Available at: http://www.netce.com/839/Course_3956.pdf. Accessed August 1, 2014.

49. Gangavati A, Hajjar I, Quach L, et al. Hypertension, orthostatic hypotension and the risk of falls in a community-dwelling elderly population: the maintenance of balance, independent living, intellect, and zest in the elderly of Boston study. J Am Geriatr Soc 2011;59:383–9. Available at: http://www.ncbi.nlm.nih.gov/pmc/articles/PMC3306056/. Accessed November 24, 2013.

50. Becker DE. Cardiovascular drugs: implications for dental practice part 1- cardiotonics, diuretics and vasodilators. Anesth Prog 2007;54:178–86 DDS2007 by the American Dental Society of Anesthesiology. p. 181. Available at: http://www.ncbi.nlm.nih.gov/pmc/articles/PMC2213250/?report=classic. Accessed November 24, 2013.

51. Aahman E, Begg S, Black B, et al. The global burden of disease: 2004 update. Geneva (Switzerland): World Health Organization; 2008. Available at: http://www.who.int/healthinfo/global_burden_disease/GBD_report_2004update_full. pdf. Accessed August 1,2014.

52. Murphy SL, Xu JQ, Kochanek KD. Deaths: final data for 2010. Natl Vital Stat Rep 2013;61(4):1–117. Available at: http://www.cdc.gov/nchs/data/nvsr/nvsr61/nvsr61_04.pdf.

53. Centers for disease control and prevention. A summary of primary stroke center policy in the United States. Atlanta (GA): U.S. Department of Health and Human Services; 2011.

54. Little JW, Falace DA, Miller CS, et al. Heart failure. In: Dental management of the medically compromised patient. Table 6-1 drugs used in the treatment of patients with heart failure. 7th edition. Missouri: Mosby; 2008. p. 81–9.

55. Bahekar AA, Singh S, Saha S, et al. The prevalence and incidence of coronary heart disease is significantly increased in peridontitis: a meta-analysis. Am Heart J 2007;154:830–7.

56. American Academy on Pediatric Dentistry Clinical Affairs Committee, American Academy on Pediatric Dentistry Council on Clinical Affairs. Guideline on antibiotic prophylaxis for dental patients at risk for infection. Pediatr Dent 2008–2009; 30(7 Suppl):215–8.

57. Richards D. Guidelines for the management of patients who are taking oral anticoagulants and who require dental surgery. Evid Based Dent 2008;9(1):5–6. http://dx.doi.org/10.1038/sj.ebd.6400558.

58. Little JW, Falace DA, Miller CS, et al. Heart failure. In: Dental management of the medically compromised patient. 7th edition. Missouri: Mosby; 2008. p. 81–9. Box 6–7.

59. Oral health topics: ultrasonis devices and cardiac pacemarkers. American Dental Association. Available at: http://www.ada.org/4933.aspx?currentTab=2. Accessed March 24, 2014.

60. Rose LF, Mealey B, Minsk L, et al. Oral care for patients with cardiovascular disease and stroke. J Am Dent Assoc 2002;133(Suppl 1):37S–44S. http://dx.doi.org/10.14219/jada.archive.2002.0378.

61. Kochanek KD, Xu JQ, Murphy SL, et al. Deaths: final data for 2009. Natl Vital Stat Rep 2011;60(3):1–116.

62. Kumar S, Selim MH, Caplan LR. Medical complications after stroke. Lancet Neurol 2010;9(1):105–18. http://dx.doi.org/10.1016/S1474-4422(09)70266-2.

63. Johnston KC, Li JY, Lyden PD, et al. Medical and neurological complications of ischemic stroke: experience from the RANTTAS trial. Stroke 1998;29(2):447–53.

64. Martino R, Foley N, Bhogal S, et al. Dysphagia after stroke: Incidence, diagnosis, and pulmonary complications. Stroke 2005;36(12):2756–63.

65. Patel M, Coshall C, Rudd AG, et al. Natural history and effects on 2-year outcomes of urinary incontinence after stroke. Stroke 2001;32:122–7.

66. Yoshida M, Murakami T, Yoshimura O, et al. The evaluation of oral health in stroke patients. Gerodontology 2012;29:e489–93.

67. Scully C, Ettinger R. The influence of systemic diseases on oral health care in older adults. J Am Dent Assoc 2007;138:7S–14S. Available at: http://jada.ada.org.

68. Arthritis Foundation. Available at: http://www.arthritis.org/conditions-treatments/understanding-arthritis/. Accessed February 23, 2014.

69. Little JW, Falace DA, Miller CS, et al. Arthritic Diseases. In: Dental management of the medically compromised patient. 6th edition. Missouri: Mosby; 2002. p. 478–500.

70. Available at: http://nihseniorhealth.gov/osteoarthritis/whatisosteoarthritis/01.html. Accessed December 5, 2013.

71. Lawrence RC, Felson DT, Helmick CG, et al. Estimates of the prevalence of arthritis and other rheumatic conditions in the United States. Part II. Arthritis Rheum 2008;58(1):26–35 [Data Source: NHANES]. Available at: http://www.ncbi.nlm.nih.gov/pmc/articles/PMC3266664/. Accessed December 6, 2013.

72. Cheng YJ, Hootman JM, Murphy LB, et al. Centers for Disease Control and Prevention (CDC). Prevalence of doctor-diagnosed arthritis and arthritis-attributable activity limitation — United States, 2007-2009. MMWR Morb Mortal Wkly Rep 2010;59(39):1261–5 [Data Source: 2007–2009 NHIS]. Available at: http://www.cdc.gov/mmwr/preview/mmwrhtml/mm5939a1.htm. Accessed December 6, 2013.

73. Srikulmontree T. Osteoarthritis. American College of Rheumatology. Available at: http://www.rheumatology.org/practice/clinical/patients/diseases_and_conditions/osteoarthritis.asp. Accessed August 1, 2014.

74. Amrein PC, Ellman L, Harris WH. Aspirin-induced prolongation of bleeding time and perioperative blood loss. J Am Med Assoc 1981;245:1825–8.

75. Ferraris VA, Swanson E. Aspirin usage and perioperative blood loss in patients undergoing unexpected operations. Surg Gynecol Obstet 1983;156:439–42.

76. NIH Consensus Development Panel on Osteoporosis Prevention, Diagnosis, and Therapy. Osteoporosis prevention, diagnosis, and therapy. JAMA 2001; 285(6):785–95.

77. WHO scientific group on the assessment of osteoporosis at primary health care level. Summary Meeting Report Brussels. Belgium, May 5–7, 2004. Available at: http://www.who.int/chp/topics/Osteoporosis.pdf.

78. Leibson CL, Toteson AN, Gabriel SE, et al. Mortality, disability, and nursing home use for persons with and without hip fracture: a population-based study. J Am Geriatr Soc 2002;50:1644–50.

79. Lamster IB, Northridge ME. Improving oral health for the elderly. New York: Springer; 2008. p. 127–56.

80. Ruggiero SL, et al. American Association of Oral and Maxillofacial Surgeons. Position paper on bisphosphonates-related osteonecrosis of the jaw- 2009 updated. Available at: http://www.aaoms.org/docs/position_papers/bronj_update.pdf. Accessed December 8, 2013.

81. Migliorati CA. Bisphosphonate-associated osteoradionecrosis: position statement. J Am Dent Assoc 2005;136:12.

82. Advisory Task Force on Bisphosphonate-Related Osteonecrosis of the Jaws, American Association of Oral and Maxillofacial Surgeons. American Association of Oral and Maxillofacial Surgeons Position Paper on Bisphosphonate-Related Osteonecrosis of the Jaws. J Oral Maxillofac Surg 2007;65:369.

83. Ruggiero SL, Dodson TB, Assael LA, et al, Task Force on Bisphosphonate-Related Osteonecrosis of the Jaws, American Association of Oral and Maxillofacial Surgeons. American Association of Oral and Maxillofacial Surgeons position paper on bisphosphonate-relate osteonecrosis of the jaw-2009 update. 2009. http://dx.doi.org/10.1111/j.1747–4477.2009.00213.x.

84. Hupp JR. Dental management of osteoporosis. C.V. Mosby; 2006. Dental Clinical Advisor. VitalBook file.

85. Woo SB, Hellstein JW, Kalmar JR. Systematyc review: bisphosphonates and osteonecrosis of the jaws. Ann Intern Med 2006;144:753–61.

Cognitive Impairment in Older Adults and Oral Health Considerations

Treatment and Management

Leonard J. Brennan, DMD[a], Jason Strauss, MD[b],*

KEYWORDS

- Cognitive impairment • Dementia • Alzheimer's disease • Rational care
- Depression • Delirium

KEY POINTS

- Worldwide incidences of degenerative cognitive diseases are increasing as the population ages. This decline in mental function frequently causes behavioral changes that directly affect oral health.
- The loss of interest and ability to complete the simple tasks of brushing and flossing can cause a rapid development of hard and soft tissue diseases that result in decreased function and increased dental pain.
- The challenge for the dental community is to understand and to identify the early signs of cognitive dysfunction so as to develop a rational treatment strategy that allows patients to comfortably maintain their teeth for as long as possible.

INTRODUCTION

Cognitive impairment is a disease or condition that presents in individuals causing them to have trouble remembering, learning new things, concentrating, or making decisions that affect their everyday life.[1] The prevalence of cognitive dysfunction increases as seniors live into their 80s and 90s.[2,3] The US Census Bureau estimated that the 2013 population of United States was 318,000,000 million people with the older than 65 segment approximately 41 million individuals. The Centers for Disease Control and Prevention (CDC) determined that of this group of 41 million seniors, 16 million suffered a broad spectrum of different cognitive dysfunctions and struggled

a Department of Oral Health Policy and Epidemiology, Harvard School of Dental Medicine, 188 Longwood Avenue, Boston, MA 02115, USA; b Geriatric Psychiatry, CHA Whidden Hospital Campus, Cambridge Health Alliance, 103 Garland Street, Everett, MA 02149, USA
* Corresponding author.
E-mail address: Jbstrauss@challiance.org

Dent Clin N Am 58 (2014) 815–828
http://dx.doi.org/10.1016/j.cden.2014.07.001
0011-8532/14/$ – see front matter © 2014 Elsevier Inc. All rights reserved.

to perform the basic activities of daily living (ADLs), including the ability to maintain good oral health (**Table 1**).[2]

Cognitive impairment is often first recognized by family and friends when a person begins to struggle with simple daily tasks.[3] Then, as the impairments increase to a more severe level, the problems with reading, writing, and understanding prevent independent living.[4] Fear of "losing one's mind" and the loss of personal control may be the single greatest worry and concern of the aging and a constant threat for everyone else.[5]

Impairment is often followed by oral health deterioration, characterized by a dramatic and quick progression of periodontal disease, caries, and tooth loss.[3,6] The process is complicated by the senior's inability to understand these changes accompanied by a loss of interest in brushing and flossing. The dentist and the dental team are called on to treat these patients in nursing homes and in office situations to maintain the patients' oral function, diagnose pathology, restore esthetics, and deliver palliative care. These impaired dental patients present to the office with confusion and frustration and unable to understand "why his gums bleed" and "asking why he has cavities."

This article on cognitive impairment discusses types and causes of cognitive impairments, the demographics of the disease in our aging population, reviews patient management protocols, and stresses the importance of using an interdisciplinary approach to delivering rational patient care.

DEMOGRAPHICS OF COGNITIVE IMPAIRMENT

In 2013, more than 70% of seniors older than 65 sought out dental care. Most of these individuals, 70%, have some of their natural teeth compared with 54% of seniors only 20 years ago. They are living in the community and are able to visit the dental office independently.[7] These older patients have successfully participated in a lifetime of prevention and treatment and feel they have "earned" their dentition. Unfortunately, as many of these individuals develop cognitive impairment problems, their motor and cognitive skills greatly diminish, resulting in a rapid progression of oral disease.[3]

In 2008, census information estimated that more than 14.5 million seniors, representing 95% of elders with cognitive impairment, live at home or in an alternate form of a living assistance program. Another 1.4 million (5%) seniors live in nursing facilities.[8–11] Cognitive impairment is the primary diagnosis for more than 68% of patients in the nursing home with an estimated 27% of the residents with mild dementia and another 41% diagnosed with severe cognitive dementia.[8–11] It is also estimated that more than 75% of the nursing home population needs daily assistance with all the ADLs, including oral health care. These individuals cannot adequately clean their teeth and often have trouble even remembering how to brush. Older adults with dementia uniformly demonstrate high levels of plaque and calculus, increased rates of caries, increased denture sores, decreased denture use, and decreased

Table 1 2013 demographics of cognition	
Estimated population of the United States	318,000,000
Estimated population older than 65	41,000,000
Estimated population older than 65 with a cognitive impairment	16,000,000

Data from Herbert LE, Scheer PA, Bienias JL, et al. Alzheimer's disease in the US population: prevalence estimates using the 2000 census. Arch Neurol 2003;60:1119–22.

salivary gland function. Additionally, any oral problems that are present before admission to the long-term care (LTC) facility tend to exacerbate once the senior is settled into the new living environment.[12]

WHAT IS A HEALTHY BRAIN AND GOOD COGNITIVE HEALTH?

The CDC defines a healthy brain as one that can perform the mental processes that are collectively known as cognition.[13] Examples of cognition are the ability to learn new things, intuition, judgment, language, and remembering. Most people think of cognitive health as staying sharp, being right in the mind, and having good genes. People from different ethnic and racial populations tend to share a core set of beliefs when they convey their thoughts on a healthy brain. Most cultures describe the activities of independent living, driving, having a good memory, and solving puzzles as a sign brain health.[13]

Public health's awareness in maintaining cognitive health is playing an important role in redefining the concept of healthy aging in today's world. Scientific studies reinforce ways to minimize risky behaviors that are related to cognitive deterioration; for example, lack of physical activity and uncontrolled high blood pressure. Even with these new lifestyle changes, normal aging, illness, and hospitalization still contribute to the decline in the ability of seniors. If cognitive dysfunction can be prevented and better treated, many older adults will enjoy a life of health and activity.

Basic self-care tasks are known as the ADLs, whereas the more complex tasks that are needed to live independently are described as instrumental ADLs (IADLs).[14] When these tasks are considered together, they help determine whether an older person can live independently (**Box 1**).[15]

Although more than 75% of residents in assisted living receive support with 1 or more ADL, 25% of the residents do not, according to a 2001 survey of assisted living communities conducted by the National Center for Assisted Living.[16] Most residents need help with oral care.

As patients with impairments progress into LTC, their ability to perform these activities continuously decreases with resulting negative behavioral changes. The prevalence of pain, mouth odor, bleeding tissues, and edentulism all increase. Studies show that the oral care that residents receive in a nursing home is poor[6] because of the lack of staff training, time constraints, and staff turnover.[12] The overall yearly retention rate in 2009 for assisted living employees was 51%. Retention rates among resident caregivers (noncertified), certified nurse assistants, and medication aides ranged from 44% to 55%.[17] By the time the caregivers are trained in the minimal basics of oral care management, many leave the facilities. Additionally, the LTC staffs are frequently asked to help manage the oral care of residents who are uncooperative, combative, and lack the ability to understand why people are invading their personal space. Rarely do these residents receive an adequate cleaning and seldom on a daily basis.[6] Unfortunately, most senior residents rely on caregivers to help maintain their oral health (**Fig. 1**).[18]

COGNITIVE IMPAIRMENT IN OLDER ADULTS
Reversible Cognitive Impairment

For older adults with cognitive difficulties, especially if this represents an abrupt change in mental status, a medical workup is always indicated to rule out a potential organic cause for this change. It is unlikely that a sudden mental status change represents a conversion to dementia. Particularly in a setting such as a hospital or a nursing home, a sudden mental status change is often the result of a delirium. Elders with

---

Box 1
Activities and the instrumental activities of daily living

Activities of daily living (ADLs) are basic self-care tasks that people usually learn in early childhood.

- Feeding
- Toileting
- Selecting proper attire
- Grooming and brushing teeth
- Maintaining continence
- Putting on clothes and bathing

Instrumental activities of daily living (IADLs) are complex skills needed to successfully live independently.

- Managing finances
- Handling transportation (driving or navigating public transit)
- Shopping
- Preparing meals
- Using the telephone and other communication devices
- Managing medications
- Housework and basic home maintenance

Data from Leon J, Lai RT. Functional status of the noninstitutionalized elderly: estimates of ADL and IADL difficulties. National Medical Expenditure Survey, research finding 4. Rockville (MD): Agency for Health Care Policy and Research, US Department of Health and Human Services; 1990. DHHS publication PHS 90–462.

Number of ADLs Supported
by Percent of Residents in Assisted Living

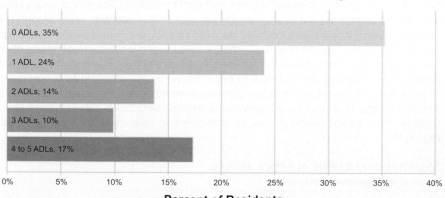

Percent of Residents

Fig. 1. Percentage of residents in assisted living requiring support. (*Data from* National Center for Assisted Living. Findings of the NCAL 2009 assisted living staff vacancy, retention and turnover survey. A NCAL study with collaboration from AAHSA, ASHA, and ALFA. Washington, DC: National Center for Assisted Living, 2010.)

delirium are characterized by inattentiveness and a fluctuating mental status. Delirious individuals may develop frightening hallucinations and become quite frightened and agitated. Delirium is most often caused by infections, electrolyte disturbances, dehydration, and medication effects and improves when the offender is treated or removed. Older adults with dementia are more vulnerable to developing delirium, and delirium is a risk factor for Alzheimer disease (AD).

Specific medical etiologies of reversible cognitive impairment may be neurologic or non-neurologic. Neurologic causes of reversible cognitive impairment can include brain lesions (ie, tumors) and normal pressure hydrocephalus, which is caused by the accumulation of cerebrospinal fluid enlarging spaces within the brain. Other medical, non-neurologic causes of reversible cognitive impairment include vitamin deficiencies (most commonly B12 deficiency), thyroid abnormalities, and neurosyphilis. All individuals receiving a workup for a change in their mental status should have vitamin B12, thyroid functioning, and rapid plasma reagin (antibodies to the organism causing syphilis) in addition to routine physical examination and laboratory work to check for these potentially reversible causes of cognitive impairment (**Table 2**).

Depression is a widespread concern in older adults, many of whom are struggling with numerous losses and life changes. Although many depressive symptoms are similar in older adults and younger adults, such as suicidal thinking, psychomotor retardation, and sleep and appetite difficulties, older adults with depression may also appear to be more withdrawn and cognitively impaired than their nondepressed counterparts. Depression in older adults may be treated with antidepressant medications and/or psychotherapy (**Box 2**).

Mild Cognitive Impairment

What differentiates mild cognitive impairment (MCI) from dementia is that the older adult experiences cognitive difficulties without a significant functional decline or impact on quality of life. Overall prevalence of MCI in the elderly is 15% to 20%, with an increased prevalence depending on age.[21] Individuals with mild cognitive impairment do not need assistance with their ADLs, such as brushing their teeth, eating, or bathing, and at most require minimal assistance with IADLs, such as taking medications, shopping for groceries, or managing finances.[22] MCI can be classified as being amnestic, nonamnestic, or of multiple domains (both amnestic and nonamnestic). Elders with amnestic MCI have particular struggles with memory and are more likely to develop Alzheimer dementia than older adults without cognitive impairment (10%–12% per year vs 1%–2% per year).[23] Older adults with nonamnestic MCI

Table 2 Reversible and irreversible dementias	
Reversible	**Irreversible**
Drugs	Alzheimer disease
Nutritional deficiencies	Multi-infarct
Normal-pressure hydrocephalous	Huntington chorea
Brain tumors	Pick disease
Hypothyroidism, hyperthyroidism	Creutzfeldt-Jakob
Neurosyphilis	Kuru
Depression	Wernicke-Korsakoff

Data from Refs.[1,7,19,20]

Box 2
Symptoms of depression

- Persistent sadness and loss of interest in the pleasures of life
- Withdrawal from society
- Weight change, insomnia, loss of appetite and energy
- Feeling of worthlessness
- Thoughts of death or suicide

Data from Caldwell P, Molloy W. Alzheimer's disease. New York: Key Porter Books; 2004.

---

struggle with other cognitive functions, such as executive functioning and aphasia. Nonamnestic MCI does not appear to reliably progress to Alzheimer dementia or other dementias. Elders with multiple-domain MCI are more likely to develop Alzheimer dementia and vascular dementia than cognitively intact peers.

Dementia

Although some of these older adults have reversible etiologies to their significant cognitive impairment, as previously stated, a vast majority of these individuals have irreversible cognitive impairment termed dementia. As noted, cognitive impairment becomes dementia when the elder develops significant functional impairment, requiring significant assistance with ADLs and IADLs. Older adults with dementia are generally unable to brush or floss. Dementia is quite common in older adults and is becoming an epidemic. Approximately 8% of all adults older than 65, 20% of individuals older than 80, and 40% of elders older than 90 have a diagnosis of dementia.[24] Although there are a great many etiologies of dementia, this article focuses on 4 of the most common causes: Alzheimer dementia, vascular dementia (VD), dementia with Lewy bodies (DLB), and frontotemporal dementia (FTD).

AD is by far the most common cause of dementia, both in the United States and worldwide.[1,2] The prevalence of AD is approximately 2% in individuals who are 65, with prevalence doubling every 5 years to a prevalence of more than 30% in adults who are 85 and older.[1,4,25–28] There is a clear genetic predisposition to AD in approximately 5% of cases,[29–35] and these individuals are more likely to develop AD earlier in life. Compared with other types of dementias, AD has an insidious onset, affecting memory, language, spatial relations, attention, and orientation, over the course of years. It is generally not until later on in the illness that personal hygiene is significantly affected.

VD is the second most commonly diagnosed form of dementia in older adults in the United States. Because their cognitive impairment is related to 1 or more cerebrovascular accidents (CVAs), individuals with VD have sensory, motor, and/or gait difficulties in addition to struggles with their memory and other cognitive functions.[1] Cognitive decline is less common in individuals with vascular dementia, occurring only with additional CVAs or the development of comorbid AD (**Fig. 2**).

A diagnosis of DLB is made when an individual develops symptoms consistent with both parkinsonism and cognitive impairment. Core diagnostic features of DLB include fluctuating attention and visual hallucinations along with parkinsonism.[1] Individuals with DLB are also quite sensitive to antipsychotic medications and may have rapid eye movement sleep behavior disorder, in which dreams are acted out, occasionally with dangerous consequences.

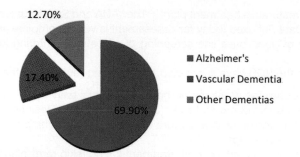

12.70%

17.40%

69.90%

■ Alzheimer's

■ Vascular Dementia

■ Other Dementias

Fig. 2. Breakdown of dementias. (*Data from* Plassman BL, Langa KM, Fisher GG, et al. Prevalence of dementia in the United States: the aging, demographics, and memory study. Neuroepidemiology 2007;29:125–32.)

Individuals with FTD are noted to have significant shrinkage of their frontal and temporal lobes. FTD is more likely to be diagnosed at a younger age[6,24,36–50] than other dementias. Memory impairment is a less prominent symptom in FTD than disinhibition, executive functioning difficulties, and overall personality changes.[51,52] Dentally, they often have noticeably poorer oral hygiene.[53–57]

MEDICAL AND DENTAL HEALTH HISTORY

The importance of a complete medical and dental history is essential to appropriately formulate a treatment plan for the patient.[38] If possible, the health history should be sent to the care providers to be completed before the dental visit. If there are any questions that need to be answered they can be researched before the patient arrives. Horowitz and Kleinman[58] suggested that having a patient or caregivers prepare a list with questions and concerns before coming to the dental office may improve dialogue and increase oral health literacy. Minimizing the transporting of a senior saves an incredible amount of patient, doctor, and caregiver time and dramatically reduces patient stress.

The additional challenge of providing the impaired with dental treatment is also complicated by the normal aging process. Declines in sensation, hearing, sight, and understanding can make the routine dental visit[59] frustrating and frightening.

EARLY INTERVENTION

Knowing that many cognitive impairment disorders are progressive, intervention in the early course of the disease is important.[6,38] Patient cooperation is often better. Patients tend to be more flexible and adaptive. For example, a patient is more apt to accept a denture or partial in the early stages of the cognitive dysfunction. Restore the teeth that can be restored and remove the teeth that will be problematic[38] while the elder patient is relatively healthy.

The importance of educating all caregivers and members of the caregiver team on the importance of diet, oral hygiene,[6] and the effect of medication on decay and periodontal disease cannot be overstressed.[39] Eating patterns and food choices are factors that affect the development of decay when sugar is inadvertently or advertently entered into a patient's diet.[60]

The American Dental Association (ADA) and Special Care Dentistry (SCD) have also recommended a new minimum data set (MDS) to evaluate patients entering nursing home facilities to detect oral disease early so as to provide a more complete preventive and restorative treatment plan.[12] The "ADA and SCD both feel that the current Minimum Data Set used today for assessment is very incomplete and emphasize the importance of good base line screening of all patients entering long term care facilities."[12]

The ADA and the SCD have suggested the following revisions to the MDS.

a. Resident has chewing problems or mouth pain/facial pain
b. Resident has abnormal mouth tissue (ulcers, masses, oral lesions)
c. Resident has a problem with a denture or partial denture (chipped, broken, loose, stained, dirty, or missing)
d. Resident has natural teeth or tooth fragments: if no, skip remaining items
e. Resident has an obvious cavity (cavities) or broken tooth (teeth)
f. Resident has a loose natural tooth (teeth)
g. Resident has inflamed bleeding gums

This information would provide measurable quantitative data for evaluating a patient's LTC and program effectiveness.[12] A thorough oral assessment would be a mechanism for early detection and treatment of oral disease. According to Guay, "the first step in solving problems understands it."[12]

OLDER ADULTS DO NOT COMMUNICATE DENTAL PROBLEMS

Senior patients do not complain about or generally discuss the dental problems that cause them stress. Rarely do they mention dental pain, a denture sore spot, or inflamed periodontal tissues. Brody[40] demonstrated that often the older patient with mild cognitive disorder frequently underreports problematic symptoms to a health care provider; 1% of 2000 symptoms were reported. The dentist must carefully ask questions and follow-up on their answers to be sure that "no pain means no pain and no problems really mean no problems."[40] Check with all caregivers to obtain information that might provide insight. With the added component of cognition, it is extremely difficult to elicit a clear picture of dental problems.

COMMUNICATION AND BEHAVIORAL STRATEGIES FOR THE COGNITIVELY IMPAIRED

Communication is challenging with an adult with cognitive impairments. Start each conversation with a self-introduction in a soft reaffirming tone and repeat if the patient becomes distracted or frightened.[41] It is important to make the patient feel secure with good eye contact, a gentle gesture, or reassuring smile. Always try to avoid patronizing talk with impaired seniors.[41] Try not to use the words "dearie" or "sweetie."[41] Patients feel less anxious if there are fewer distractions in the operatory, people included, when treatment is initiated.[42]

The use of a nonpharmacological approach in treating patients should be used whenever possible.[53] Pharmacologic management can be an important tool, but should be used cautiously because they can elicit adverse and variable effects on individuals.[43,44]

As stated by Kovach,[43] "people with dementias are heterogeneous in disability, clinical course, and treatment success" and interventions will work for some and not for others with dementia, and what works today for one person may no longer be effective next week or month. If a cognitively impaired patient has behavioral problems, they are usually the reaction of the individual to an interaction with the physical environment, social environment, and dementia management issue (**Box 3**).[4,46,61]

The dental team needs to learn strategies to improve communication with seniors. Doing so will enable providers to deliver the best care with optimum health

---

Box 3
Effective communication strategies for the cognitively impaired adults

Appointment Strategies for the cognitively impaired patient

Before the appointment

   Schedule longer appointment times

   Ask patients to prepare and bring a written list of questions to the appointment

During the appointment

   Provide a warm greeting

   Sit face-to-face with the patient

   Maintain appropriate eye contact

   Ask open-ended questions, such as "What are your concerns today?"

   Listen attentively (and limit distractions)

   Use simple language (and avoid medical jargon)

   Speak slowly, clearly, and loudly (but do not use a patronizing tone)

   Present the most important points first

   Present points one at a time

   Ask the patient to repeat the provider's most important points

   Use visual aids when possible

After the appointment

   Provide written instructions for the patient to review at home

   Follow-up with a telephone call to check on the patient's condition in cases of extractions, implants, root canal therapy, large restorations, or other complex procedures

Data from DeWalt DA, Callahan LF, Hawk VH, et al. Health literacy universal precautions toolkit (prepared by North Carolina Network Consortium, The Cecil G. Sheps Center for Health Services Research, The University of North Carolina at Chapel Hill). Rockville (MD): Agency for Healthcare Research and Quality; 2010. AHRQ publication 10–0046-EF. Available at: www.ahrq.gov/professionals/quality-patient-safety/quality-resources/tools/literacy-toolkit/index.html. Accessed January 3, 2014.

---

outcomes.[45] In a national survey conducted by Rozier and colleagues,[45] they found that most dentists do not feel that dental school prepared them with the skills needed to communicate with elder patients and are unsure on how to best approach a senior patient.

TREATMENT PLANNING CONSIDERATIONS AND RATIONAL CARE FOR THE COGNITIVELY IMPAIRED

There is a commonality in providing dental treatment for the cognitively impaired. After a patient is diagnosed with impairment, it is important for the dentist to begin early intervention.[62] As patients transition from mild to severe disease, they become increasing more difficult to manage behaviorally and dentally. In later stages of the disease, patients do not comprehend or trust the treatment activities in an office. At first diagnosis, a unified approach to care needs to be developed. It is important to take into consideration the patient's personal abilities, skill levels, and interest in home care before designing a treatment plan.[63] Other factors that may influence decision-making include social, economic, financial, family, medical, and transportation issues.[63,64] Successful care of adults is not task oriented but is centered on the needs of the patient.[64] Hallberg further emphasized that "Care that is poorly adapted to a patient's needs, leads to the emergence of behavior that is disruptive."[65]

Planning treatment and managing care for an elderly patient can be complicated.[66] As patients age and their physical and mental health deteriorates, dentists are continuously challenged to alter treatment plans to accommodate these changes.[67] An elderly patient may not be able to tolerate extensive restorative procedures, and often it may be necessary to shorten and redefine achievable goals for each appointment.[63]

The Canadian Dental Association's Committee on Clinical and Scientific Affairs produced an excellent document on rational dental care for the cognitively impaired elderly patients for seniors that are homebound and living in LTC facilities. The importance of prevention is stressed. The article emphasizes the following[64]:

1. Establishing good preventive technique while the older patient is still relatively healthy.
2. Diet education, hygiene education, and patient-specific measures to increase tooth resistance is of primary importance.
3. Rational dental care individualized to a patient's needs.
4. Individualized treatment protocol for the patient that take into consideration the person's ability to handle stress, and reasonable treatments that are less extensive.
5. Consider the ability of a patient to maintain dental treatment.

Good evidence exists that oral health care can influence the quality of life of all seniors[36,68,69] while preventing oral diseases.[67]

THE IMPORTANCE OF USING AN INTERDISCIPLINARY APPROACH IN PROVIDING DENTAL TREATMENT FOR THE COGNITIVELY IMPAIRED PATIENT

Caring for cognitively impaired patients requires the bringing together of an interdisciplinary team of family members, dentist, hygienists, physicians, pharmacist, and other care supporters to provide support and determine the treatment protocols. The interdisciplinary model may provide the most complete working example for successfully treating seniors.[70] Individuals of different disciplines need to collaborate in developing the best treatment plan for the patient and then continuously communicate and monitor progress. For example, all of the team needs to be educated on the effect of diet, xerostomia, and pharmacology on caries and periodontal disease. It is equally important that the entire disciplinary team understand the direction and goals of the dental treatment plan.[70]

SUMMARY

As the population of the United States ages, the prevalence of many cognitive dysfunction syndromes increases. It is important for the dental team to understand and recognize the early signs of the disease and to be aware that the behavioral changes caused by dementia profoundly affect the oral environment.[6] The deterioration of the oral hard and soft tissue often progress rapidly into periodontal disease, tooth decay, tooth loss, sore tissues, and pain. The involvement of the entire interdisciplinary team supports the best dental care management for the patient.

Early intercession provides the elder with treatment that maximizes function and minimizes the stress associated with oral disease. Dental treatment plans need to be developed to a patient's level of functioning, life expectancy, comorbidities, and personal goals. As a patient progresses from a mild to a more severe cognitive impairment, goals need to be reassessed and changed appropriately. Then, in conjunction with the patient's interdisciplinary team, a rational, workable and effective treatment plan can be flexibly developed.

REFERENCES

1. Lamster IB, Northridge ME. Improving oral health for the elderly. New York: Springer; 2008.
2. Herbert LE, Scherr PA, Bienias JL, et al. Alzheimer disease in the US population: prevalence estimates using the 2000 census. Arch Neurol 2003;60:1119–22.
3. Papas AS, Niessen LC, Chauncey HH. Geriatric dentistry: aging and oral health. St Louis (MO): Mosby; 1991.
4. Kaplan HI, Sadock BJ, Grebb JA. Kaplan and Sadock's synopsis of psychiatry: behavioral sciences, clinical psychiatry. 7th edition. Baltimore (MD): Williams & Wilkins; 1994.
5. Research! America. America speaks: poll data summary, vol. 7. Alexandria (Egypt): Research! America; 2006. p. 25–6. Available at: http://www.researchamerica.org/uploads/americaspeaksv7.pdf.
6. Chalmers J, Pearson A. Oral hygiene care for residents with dementia: a literature review. J Adv Nurs 2005;52:410–9.
7. Mooyman N, Kiyak HA. Social gerontology: a multidisciplinary perspective. Needham Heights (MA); 1988. Allyn & Bacon.
8. Murtaugh CM, Freiman MP. Nursing home residents at risk of hospitalization and the characteristics of their hospital stays. Gerontologist 1995;35(1):35–43.
9. Murtaugh CM, Kemper P, Spillman BC. The risk of nursing home use in later life. Med Care 1990;28(10):952–62.
10. Murtaugh CM, Kemper P, Spillman BC. Risky business: long-term care insurance underwriting. Inquiry 1995;32:271–84.
11. Murtaugh CM, Kemper P, Spillman BC, et al. The amount, distribution and timing of lifetime nursing home use. Med Care 1995;35(3):204–18.
12. Guay AH. The oral health status of nursing home residents: what we need to know? J Dent Educ 2005;69(9):1015–7.
13. Anderson L, Logsdon RG, Hochhalter AK, et al. Introduction to the special issue on promoting cognitive health in diverse populations of older adults. Gerontologist 2009;49(Suppl 1):S1–2.
14. Leon J, Lai RT. Functional status of the noninstitutionalized elderly: estimates of ADL and IADL difficulties. National Medical Expenditure Survey, research finding 4. Rockville (MD): Agency for Health Care Policy and Research, U.S. Department of Health and Human Services; 1990. DHHS publication PHS 90–3462.
15. Spector WD, Katz S, Murphy JB, et al. The hierarchical relationship between activities of daily living and instrumental activities of daily living. J Chronic Dis 1987;40:481–90.
16. Wivel ME. NIMH report. NIH consensus conference stresses need to identify reversible causes of dementia. Hosp Community Psychiatry 1988;39:22–3.
17. ALSA, ASAH, AANSA, CAL, NIC FINDINGS OF THE NCAL 2009. Assisted living staff vacancy, retention and turnover survey. Survey 2009. Available at: http://www.ahcancal.org/ncal/quality/Documents/.
18. Chalmers JM, Levy SM, Buckwalter KC, et al. Factors influencing nurses' aides' provisions of oral care for nursing facility residents. Spec Care Dentist 1996; 16(2):71–9.
19. Fenstemacher PA, Winn P. Long-term care medicine, vol. 11. New York: Humana Press; 2011. p. 236–43.

20. Flaherty JH. Psychotherapeutic agents in older adults. Commonly prescribed and over-the-counter remedies: causes of confusion. Clin Geriatr Med 1998; 14:101–27.
21. Lopez OL, Jagust WJ, DeKosky SI, et al. Prevalence and classification of mild cognitive impairment in the Cardiovascular Health Study Cognition Study: part 1. Arch Neurol 2003;60:1385–9.
22. Forlenza OV, Diniz BS, Stella F, et al. Mild cognitive impairment (part 1): clinical characteristics and predictors of dementia. Rev Bras Psiquiatr 2013;35: 178–85.
23. Peterson RC, Doody R, Kurz A, et al. Current concepts in mild cognitive impairment. Arch Neurol 2001;58:1985–92.
24. Ferri CP, Prince M, Brayne C, et al. Global prevalence of dementia: a Delphi consensus study. Lancet 2005;366:2112–7.
25. Kokmen E, Beard CM, O'Brien PC, et al. Is the incidence of dementing illness changing? A 25-year time trend study in Rochester, Minnesota (1960–1984). Neurology 1993;43:1887–92.
26. Drachman DA. If we live long enough, will we all be demented? Neurology 1994; 44:1563–665.
27. Rowe JW. Health care of the elderly. N Engl J Med 1985;312:827–35.
28. Minaker KL, Rowe J. Health and disease among the oldest old: a clinical perspective. Milbank Mem Fund Q Health Soc 1985;63:324–49.
29. Silverman JM, Ciresi G, Smith CJ, et al. Variability of familial risk of Alzheimer disease across the late life span. Arch Gen Psychiatry 2005;62(5):565–73.
30. Frenkel H. Alzheimer's disease and oral care. Dent Update 2004;31(5):273–4, 276–8.
31. Gustafson L, Nilsson L. Differential diagnosis of prehensile dementia on clinical grounds. Acta Psychiatr Scand 1982;65:194–209.
32. American Psychiatric Association. Diagnostic and statistical manual of mental disorders. 4th edition. Washington, DC: American Psychiatric Association; 1994.
33. Campbell S, Stephens S, Ballard C. Dementia with Lewy bodies: clinical features and treatment. Drugs Aging 2001;18:397–407.
34. McKeith IG. Spectrum of Parkinson's disease, Parkinson's dementia, and Lewy body dementia. Neurol Clin 2000;18:865–902.
35. Serby M, Samuels SC. Diagnostic criteria for dementia with Lewy bodies reconsidered. Am J Geriatr Psychiatry 2001;9:212–6.
36. Spitzer WO. State of science 1986: quality of life and functional status as target variables for research. J Chronic Dis 1987;40:465–71.
37. MacEntee MI. Quality of life as an indicator of oral health in older people. J Am Dent Assoc 2007;138(9 Suppl):47S–52S.
38. Chalmers JM. Minimal intervention dentistry: part 2. Strategies for addressing restorative challenges in older patients. J Can Dent Assoc 2006;72(5): 435–40.
39. Burt BA. Epidemiology of dental diseases in the elderly. Clin Geriatr Med 1992; 8(3):59.
40. Brody EM. Tomorrow and tomorrow and tomorrow: toward squaring the suffering curve. In: Gaitz CM, Niederebe G, Wilson NL, editors. Aging 2000. New York, NY: Springer-Verlag; 1985. p. 371–80.
41. DeWalt DA, Callahan LF, Hawk VH, et al. Health Literacy Universal Precautions Toolkit (prepared by North Carolina Network Consortium, The Cecil G. Sheps Center for Health Services Research, The University of North Carolina at Chapel Hill). Rockville (MD): Agency for Healthcare Research and Quality; 2010. AHRQ publication

10-0046-EF. Available at: www.ahrq.gov/professionals/quality-patient-safety/quality-resources/tools/literacy-toolkit/index.html. Accessed January 3, 2014.

42. Kayser-Jones J, Bird WF, Redford M, et al. Strategies for conducting dental examinations among cognitively impaired nursing home residents. Spec Care Dentist 1996;16(2):46–52.

43. Kovach CR. Late stage dementia care: a basic guide. Washington, DC: Taylor & Francis; 1997.

44. Friedlander AH, Jarvik LF. The dental management of patients with dementia. Oral Surg Oral Med Oral Pathol 1987;64:549–53.

45. Rozier GR, Horowitz AM, Podschun G. Dentist-patient communication techniques used in the United States: the results of a national survey. J Am Dent Assoc 2011;142(5):518–30.

46. Jablonski RA, Therrien B, Mahoney EK, et al. An intervention to reduce care-resistant behavior in persons with dementia during oral hygiene: a pilot study. Spec Care Dentist 2011;31(3):77–87.

47. Fick DM, Agostini JV, Inouye SK. Delirium superimposed on dementia: a systems review. J Am Geriatr Soc 2002;50:1723–32.

48. Petersen RC, O'Brien J. Mild cognitive impairment should be considered for DSM-V. J Geriatr Psychiatry Neurol 2006;19:147–54.

49. Morris JC. Mild cognitive impairment is early-stage Alzheimer disease: time to revise diagnostic criteria. Arch Neurol 2006;63:15–6.

50. Petersen RC, Smith GE, Waring SC, et al. Mild cognitive impairment: clinical characterization and outcome. Arch Neurol 1999;56:303–8.

51. McKhann GM, Albert MS, Grossman M, et al. Clinical and pathological diagnosis of frontotemporal dementia: a report of the Work Group on Frontotemporal and Pick's Disease. Arch Neurol 2001;58:1803–9.

52. Bozeat S, Gregory CA, Ralph MA, et al. Which neuropsychiatric and behavioral features distinguish frontal and temporal variants of frontotemporal dementias from Alzheimer's disease? J Neurol Neurosurg Psychiatr 2000;69:178–86.

53. Kertesz A, Munoz DG. Frontotemporal dementia. Med Clin North Am 2002;86:501–18.

54. Binetti G, Locascio JJ, Corkin S, et al. Differences between Pick disease and Alzheimer's disease in clinical appearance and rate of cognitive decline. Arch Neurol 2000;57:225–32.

55. Clarfield AM. The decreasing prevalence of reversible dementias: an updated meta-analysis. Arch Intern Med 2003;163:2219–29.

56. American Medical Directors Association. Delirium and acute problematic behavior in the long-term care setting clinical practice guidelines. Columbia (MD): AMDA; 2008.

57. Inouye SK. Delirium in older persons. N Engl J Med 2006;354:1157–65.

58. Horowitz AM, Kleinman DV. Creating a health literacy-based practice. J Calif Dent Assoc 2012;40(4):331–40.

59. Stein PS, Aalboe JA, Savage MW, et al. Strategies for communicating with older dental patients. J Am Dent Assoc 2014;145(2):159–64.

60. Chauncey HH, Epstein S, Rose C, et al. Clinical geriatric dentistry: biomedical and psychological aspect. Chicago: ADA; 1985.

61. Chalmers JM. Behavior management and communication strategies for dental professionals when caring for patients with dementia. Spec Care Dentist 2000;20(4):147–54.

62. Ettinger RL. Rational dental care: part 1. Has the concept changed in 20 years? J Can Dent Assoc 2006;72(5):441–5.

63. Ettinger RL. Clinical decision-making in the treatment of elderly. Gerontology 1984;3(2):157–65.
64. CDA Committee on Clinical and Scientific Affairs. Best practices for aging adults in private practice. Dent Assist 2012;81(1):38.
65. Hallberg IR, Holst G, Nordmark A, et al. Cooperation during morning care between nurses and severely demented institutionalized patients. Clin Nurs Res 1995;4:78–104.
66. Lindquist TJ, Ettinger RL. The complexities involved with managing the care of an elderly patient. J Am Dent Assoc 2003;134(5):593–600.
67. Berkley DB, Berg RG, Ettinger RL, et al. The old-old dental patient: the challenge of clinical decision making. J Am Dent Assoc 1996;127(3):321–32.
68. Family Caregiver Alliance. Available at: www.caregiver.org/caregiver/jsp/content_node.jsp?nodeid=438. Accessed January 21, 2014.
69. Otsuni E, Mohl G. Communicating more effectively with the confused or demented patient. Gen Dent 1995;43:264–6.
70. Satin DS. Health management for older adults: developing an interdisciplinary approach. New York: Oxford; 2009.

Integrating Oral Health into the Interdisciplinary Health Sciences Curriculum

Maria C. Dolce, PhD, RN, CNE[a],*, Nona Aghazadeh-Sanai, DDS[b],
Shan Mohammed, MD, MPH[c], Terry T. Fulmer, PhD, RN[d,e]

KEYWORDS

- Collaborative practice • Interprofessional education • Oral health
- Team-based competencies

KEY POINTS

- The burden of oral diseases and access to care are significant health challenges for an aging society, and calls for reforms in health professions education.
- Transformation of health professions education necessitates innovative models linking interprofessional education (IPE) and collaborative practice.
- Innovations in Interprofessional Oral Health: Technology, Instruction, Practice, Service is an innovative IPE model for integrating oral health in health sciences curricula.
- The Program of All-inclusive Care for the Elderly (PACE) is a patient-centered interdisciplinary practice model for improving oral health of older adults.

INTRODUCTION

Over the last 100 years there has been a historical movement of change in the landscape of professional health education in North America. Seminal reports, such as Flexner (1910),[1] Welch and Rose (1915),[2] Goldmark (1923),[3] and Gies (1926),[4] influenced instructional and institutional reforms in medicine, public health, nursing, and

Funding Sources: DentaQuest Foundation (M.C. Dolce).
Conflict of Interest: The authors have nothing to disclose.
[a] School of Nursing, Bouvé College of Health Sciences, Northeastern University, 310 Robinson Hall, 360 Huntington Avenue, Boston, MA 02115, USA; [b] Department of Oral Health Policy and Epidemiology, Harvard School of Dental Medicine, 188 Longwood Avenue, Boston, MA 02115, USA; [c] Department of Health Sciences, Bouvé College of Health Sciences, Northeastern University, 312C Robinson Hall, 360 Huntington Avenue, Boston, MA 02115, USA; [d] School of Nursing, Bouvé College of Health Sciences, Northeastern University, 215 Behrakis Health Sciences Center, 360 Huntington Avenue, Boston, MA 02115, USA; [e] Public Policy and Urban Affairs, College of Social Sciences and Humanities, Northeastern University, 360 Huntington Avenue, Boston, MA 02115, USA
* Corresponding author.
E-mail address: m.dolce@neu.edu

dentistry. These early reports generated groundbreaking shifts toward advancing scientific curricula, linking education to research, and establishing professional education in universities. In 2010, the Lancet Commission,[5] a global independent Commission on Education of Health Professionals for the twenty-first century, assessed educational institutions in medicine, nursing, and public health from global and systems perspectives. Despite a century of reforms, professional health education had not kept pace with global health challenges and inequities, shifts in societal demographics and burden of diseases, advances in scientific knowledge and technology, and increasing complexity of health care systems.

Oral health is a neglected global and local health issue, and the burden of oral diseases has significant consequences for individuals, populations, and health systems worldwide.[6] In 2012, there were approximately 810 million people aged 60 or older, and this number is projected to increase to more than 2 billion by 2050.[7] Given the trend in global population aging, improving oral health and general health for an aging society presents an immense challenge. More than a decade ago, the US Surgeon General described the nation's poor oral health status as a "silent epidemic" and brought widespread attention to the vast oral health inequities that persist today.[8] Although overall improvements in oral health have been reported, the burden of oral disease and access to oral health care remain significant for vulnerable and underserved populations, particularly older Americans.[8–10] Several factors contribute to poor oral health care for older adults, including inadequate education of nondental health care professionals (eg, nurses, pharmacists, physicians, and others) about oral health and diseases, and the lack of attention to oral health by health care professionals.[8–10] Moreover, health professionals and dental professionals have been educated separately, thus promoting the separation of oral health from general health.[9,10] Academic institutions need to enhance curricula to address the global challenges of oral health and local oral health care needs of an aging population.

The transformation of professional health education to strengthen the performance of health systems in meeting the needs of patients and populations is an imperative for academic institutions.[5] Curricular reforms are needed to effectually respond to local and global health contexts and advance health equity for individuals and populations.[5] The Lancet Commission provides a framework for action through its proposed set of academic reforms for the next century, including the adoption of a competency-based approach to curricula, promotion of interprofessional education (IPE), and application of advanced technologies for professional health education.[5]

Advancing oral health warrants bold action from educational institutions, and necessitates new models of IPE that are responsive to global and local oral health needs of an aging society. This article discusses the Bouvé College of Health Sciences (Bouvé College) at Northeastern University's response to the call to action for transforming professional health education, and describes its IPE model for strengthening the primary care health system to promote healthy aging. The Innovations in Interprofessional Oral Health: Technology, Instruction, Practice and Service (Oral Health TIPS) program at Bouvé College is an innovative IPE model that aims to prepare the next generation of health professionals with requisite team-based competencies to meet the oral and systemic health needs of vulnerable and underserved patients and populations, particularly older adults. Mechanisms for integrating oral health into interdisciplinary health sciences curricula are described. The discussion concludes with an exemplar case for aligning IPE and clinical practice to improve oral and systemic health outcomes for older adults in a patient-centered medical home.

BACKGROUND AND SIGNIFICANCE
Oral Health Call-to-Action

In 2000, the US Surgeon General's report, *Oral Health in America*, raised awareness about the importance of good oral health as an integral component of general health and well-being.[8] The report highlighted the potential contribution of all health care professions to improve oral health, and the necessity for collaborative, interdisciplinary approaches to care. With appropriate education in oral health promotion and disease prevention, primary care providers are well positioned to integrate oral health as a component of general health.[8] The report presented a framework for action to address oral health inequities and optimize the oral and general health care systems. Preparing health professionals with the competencies to collaborate with each other in providing oral health care as a component of comprehensive care requires curricula reform with an increased emphasis on interdisciplinary training.[8] In 2003, a partnership of public and private organizations issued a national call to action to enable further progress in improving oral health.[11] The need to revise curricula and include interdisciplinary training were reiterated as important actions to enhance the capacity of all health professionals in improving access to oral health care.[11] In 2011, the Institute of Medicine (IOM) released two independent reports, *Advancing Oral Health in America*,[10] and *Improving Access to Oral Health Care for Vulnerable and Underserved Populations*.[9] Although some improvements have been reported in the last decade, vulnerable and underserved populations in the United States continue to suffer the burden and consequences of oral diseases.[9] Both reports underscored the pivotal role of all health care professionals in oral health promotion and disease prevention, the value of interprofessional team-based care to improve oral health, and the need for additional education and training of health professionals in oral health.[9,10]

IPE for Collaborative Practice and Teamwork

IPE for collaborative practice and teamwork has been an important and enduring movement in health care.[12] **Box 1** provides a description of terms.[13,14] Early work in

---

Box 1
Description of terms

Interprofessional education "occurs when two or more professions learn about, from and with each other to enable effective collaboration and improve health outcomes."[13]

Collaborative practice "occurs when multiple health workers from different professional backgrounds provide comprehensive services by working with patients, their families, carers and communities to deliver the highest quality of care across settings."[13]

Interprofessional teamwork is "the levels of cooperation, coordination and collaboration characterizing the relationships between professions in delivering patient-centered care."[14]

Interprofessional competencies in health care refers to the "integrated enactment of knowledge, skills, and values/attitudes that define working together across the professions, with other health care workers, and with patients, along with families and communities, as appropriate to improve health outcomes in specific care contexts."[14]

Adapted from World Health Organization Study Group on Interprofessional Education and Collaborative Practice. Framework for action on interprofessional education and collaborative practice. Geneva (Switzerland): World Health Organization; 2010. Available at: http://whqlibdoc.who.int/hq/2010/WHO_HRH_HPN_10.3_eng.pdf; and Interprofessional Education Collaborative Expert Panel. Core competencies for interprofessional collaborative practice: a report of an expert panel. Washington, DC: Interprofessional Education Collaborative; 2011. Available at: http://www.aacn.nche.edu/education-resources/ipecreport.pdf.

IPE and team training in the United States can be traced to 1969, with the institution of an interdisciplinary health sciences curriculum at the University of Nevada School of Medical Sciences aimed at promoting teamwork in primary care.[15] Contemporary dialogue on interdisciplinary team-based education for US health professions was signaled by the 1972 IOM conference, "Interrelationships of Educational Programs for Health Professionals."[15] This pioneering event convened 120 leaders from five health professions (allied health, dentistry, medicine, nursing, and pharmacy) to explore the promises and challenges of educating for teamwork in health care.[15] These leaders recommended that the educational process should not isolate students in the health professions from each other, and interdisciplinary education should be linked to practice needs in health care systems.[15] In the twenty-first century, a resurgence of the IPE movement in the United States was marked by its national focus on health care quality and patient safety. In 2003, the IOM landmark report, *Health Professions Education: A Bridge to Quality*, impressed the need for IPE and collaborative practice to improve health care quality and safety, and recommended teamwork as a core interprofessional competency for all health professionals.[16]

In 2010, the World Health Organization issued its global *Framework for Action on Interprofessional Education and Collaborative Practice* to strengthen the health system and improve health outcomes through effective training in collaborative teamwork.[13] The global aim is to develop a "collaborative practice-ready" workforce (ie, students ready to enter the health care system as members of a collaborative practice team).[13] The 2010 Lancet Commission report underscored the importance of teamwork as a cross-cutting competency for all health professions and led to the formation of the IOM Global Forum on Innovation in Health Professional Education.[5,17] This forum brings together leaders from academia, professional associations, and government to advance the global discourse on health profession education through institutional and instructional reform. In 2011, the US Interprofessional Education Collaborative (IPEC) Expert Panel, comprised of members from the American Association of Colleges of Nursing, Association of American Medical Colleges, American Dental Education Association, Association of Schools of Public Health, and American Association of Colleges of Osteopathic Medicine, established core competencies for interprofessional collaborative practice.[14] The IPEC core competency domains are described in **Box 2**.

Box 2
Core competencies for interprofessional collaborative practice

Values/ethics for interprofessional practice: "Work with individuals of other professions to maintain a climate of mutual respect and shared values."

Roles and responsibilities for collaborative practice: "Use the knowledge of one's own role and those of other professions to appropriately assess and address the healthcare needs of the patients and populations served."

Interprofessional communication practices: "Communicate with patients, families, communities, and other health professionals in a responsive and responsible manner that supports a team approach to the maintenance of health and the treatment of disease."

Interprofessional teamwork and team-based practice: "Apply relationship-building values and the principles of team dynamics to perform effectively in different team roles to plan and deliver patient-/population-centered care that is safe, timely, efficient, effective, and equitable."

Adapted from Interprofessional Education Collaborative Expert Panel. Core competencies for interprofessional collaborative practice: a report of an expert panel. Washington, DC: Interprofessional Education Collaborative; 2011. Available at: http://www.aacn.nche.edu/education-resources/ipecreport.pdf.

Connecting Dental and Health Sciences through Innovations

In response to the 2003 IOM report,[16] New York University (NYU) demonstrated bold action by creating an innovative institutional partnership model that organized the College of Nursing within the College of Dentistry.[18,19] Initiated in 2005 under the visionary leadership of Drs Michael Alfano and Terry Fulmer, this unique interdisciplinary model cultivated vast opportunities for interprofessional collaborations in research, education, and practice. Nursing and dental students learned about, from, and with each other, in a variety of IPE experiences including didactics, clinic rotations, global outreach, and community service. Evidence-based practice was a major curricular theme and cross-cutting competency, which served to advance IPE across the dental and nursing programs. Importantly, dental and nursing students learned about each other's professional roles and contributions to improve oral and systemic health through evidence-based care.

The institutional model at NYU continues to generate innovations in interprofessional collaboration, such as the establishment of a nurse practitioner–managed primary care practice colocated at the College of Dentistry.[18,20] This interprofessional practice model resulted in cross-referrals between primary care and dental clinics, and the integration of oral health as a component of comprehensive health in a nurse practitioner–managed primary care clinic. In 2011, a distinct interprofessional curriculum, NYU3T: Teaching, Technology, Teamwork, was implemented at the NYU College of Nursing and School of Medicine.[21] The NYU3T curriculum was grounded in two evidence-based team training programs: Geriatric Interdisciplinary Team Training[22] and TeamSTEPPS.[23] This innovative program exploits the novel use of collaborative online learning, virtual patient cases, and simulation-learning to enhance team-based competencies.[21]

Another outcome of this innovative academic partnership is the Oral Health Nursing Education and Practice program, which was launched in 2011.[24] This national program aimed to prepare a collaborative practice-ready nursing workforce with the competencies to prioritize oral health promotion and disease prevention, provide oral health care in a variety of practice settings, and collaborate in interprofessional teams to improve access to oral health care.[24] The innovative synergies created at NYU served as a catalyst for expanding oral health education across all health sciences curricula at Bouvé College.

Bouvé College

Bouvé College is an innovative, and contemporary educational institution uniquely poised to advance IPE in health sciences under the new leadership of Dean Terry Fulmer, formerly the founding Dean of NYU College of Nursing. Bouvé College is the largest health sciences college in metropolitan Boston with more than 3700 students, 186 full-time faculty, and 145 part-time faculty within its three schools: Health Professions, Nursing, and Pharmacy. The School of Health Professions is comprised of four academic departments (Counseling and Applied Educational Psychology, Health Sciences, Physical Therapy, and Speech-Language Pathology and Audiology) and a Physician Assistant program. The School of Nursing has both baccalaureate and graduate programs. The School of Pharmacy consists of two departments: Pharmaceutical Sciences and Pharmacy Practice. Bouvé College has three interdisciplinary programs (biotechnology, health informatics, and personal health informatics) and 10 interdisciplinary research centers within the University.

Health is one of three strategic areas of commitment at Northeastern University, and Bouvé College is setting the standard for excellence in innovations, research, education, and practice. The mission of Bouvé College is to inspire and create the next generation of interprofessional health care leaders for the well-being of our global community. Students are prepared for interprofessional practice through campus-based learning and experiential education. Bouvé College is at the vanguard of improving health through its four pillars of excellence: (1) Drug Discovery, Delivery, and Diagnostics; (2) Urban Population Health; (3) Self-care/Self-management; and (4) Healthy Aging. This framework provides a platform for interdisciplinary partnerships in research, teaching, and practice within Bouvé College, across the University, and between other academic institutions and health systems. Bouvé College continues to expand its dedicated cluster of faculty focused on advancing the science of healthy aging and team-based geriatric care.

Bouvé College envisions a new generation of interprofessional health care leaders with team-based competencies to improve oral health and healthy aging across the life cycle, particularly for vulnerable and underserved populations. This goal requires a fundamental shift in health sciences curricula and care delivery models to enhance the integration of oral health care as an essential component of comprehensive primary health care, with an emphasis on oral health promotion and prevention. Every primary care visit is an opportunity for clinicians to incorporate oral health into their practice.[25] Nurses, nurse practitioners, pharmacists, physicians, physician assistants, and other health professionals can address oral health promotion and prevention as a component of comprehensive health in a variety of primary care settings including private offices, community health centers, retail medical clinics, and pharmacies. To that end, Bouvé College is making great advances in integrating oral health education in interdisciplinary health sciences curricula through its innovative IPE program, Oral Health TIPS, funded by the DentaQuest Foundation and launched in 2013. The purpose of the Oral Health TIPS model is to enhance the capacity of the primary care health system for improving oral health across the life cycle, particularly for vulnerable and underserved populations.

ORAL HEALTH TIPS
Program Overview

Equipping faculty and graduates with the knowledge, skills, and attitudes to integrate oral health promotion and oral disease prevention into practice, and shifting from educating health professionals separately to team-based education are high priorities at Bouvé College. The overarching goal of the Oral Health TIPS program is to prepare primary care professionals across disciplines with team-based competencies to integrate oral health into comprehensive general health care, with an emphasis on health promotion and disease prevention. The primary aims of the program are to integrate oral health education across interdisciplinary health sciences curricula; and promote team-based, collaborative practice models for oral health promotion and disease prevention in primary care settings. The Oral Health TIPS program builds on the collaborative work of the National Interprofessional Initiative on Oral Health, whose mission is to engage primary care clinicians in oral health.[26]

Approach

Organizational leadership is paramount in transforming health professions education to address local and global oral health challenges. The Oral Health TIPS program is supported by a multilevel leadership infrastructure that includes deans, directors, faculty, and students across Bouvé College and its Schools of Health Professions, Nursing, and Pharmacy. Organizational engagement strategies include convening discussion forums and presentations to create awareness about oral health inequities, align faculty and students toward a shared vision of improving oral health through interprofessional collaborative practice, and make the case for integrating oral health as an essential component of comprehensive health care in primary care settings. Faculty members from each academic department serve as oral health champions and facilitators for integrating oral health and teamwork competencies into their respective health science curriculum.

The Oral Health TIPS program uses a multimodal approach to advance IPE and collaborative practice in oral health. Learning innovations bring students together from multiple health professions to learn about, from, and with each other. Interprofessional learning is contextualized using a team-based approach to improving oral health and promoting healthy aging across the life cycle. The approach integrates strategies for adopting competency-based curricula, strengthening educational resources, promoting team-based practice, leveraging educational technologies, and designing experiential learning.

Adopting competency-based curricula
The IPEC core competencies for interprofessional collaborative practice[18] are adopted as a framework for advancing the integration of oral health into health sciences curricula, and preparing graduates with basic oral health competencies to assess risk for oral diseases, provide oral health promotion and disease prevention information, integrate oral health information with patient and family counseling about healthy personal behaviors, and make referrals to dentists and other health professionals.[9] *Smiles for Life: A National Oral Health Curriculum*[27] is endorsed as an online, modular curriculum for integration into existing undergraduate and graduate courses across the health sciences. For example, Course 8: Geriatric Oral Health addresses the role of primary care clinicians in promoting oral health for older adults through comprehensive oral assessments and collaborating with dental professionals. Faculty can readily integrate this module in courses that address the management of common geriatric oral-systemic health problems.

Strengthening educational resources
Strengthening educational resources is essential to enhance oral health and teamwork competencies.[5] The Oral Health TIPS program prioritizes faculty development through investing in ongoing train-the-trainer workshops and other educational programs designed to enhance oral health and team-based competencies. The *Smiles for Life* curriculum is featured as a strategy for faculty enrichment.[28] Faculty development programs focus on integrating oral health care into comprehensive primary health care, common oral-systemic health problems, oral health promotion and disease prevention for healthy aging, and the medical-dental interface. The Dean's Seminar Series offers faculty and students the opportunity to learn about current issues in oral and systemic health, and engage in conversational learning with prominent leaders in research, education, practice, and policy.

Promoting team-based practice
Adopting teamwork as a cross-cutting competency for all health professionals, the Oral Health TIPS program uses team-based instructional methods to prepare students for effective team-based practice. Instructional methods are designed to engage students from multiple professions to learn together, particularly about each other's roles; work toward a common goal; and collaborate across traditional professional boundaries. Collaborative didactic teaching-learning, specially designed to enhance core competencies for collaborative practice, is an effective strategy for

engaging students across health professions to learn about, from, and with each other toward a shared goal of improving oral-systemic health in a primary care setting. For example, faculty from Bouvé College, Harvard School of Dental Medicine, and Harvard Medical School collaborated on the design, planning, and implementation of IPE didactic sessions at the Beth Israel Deaconess Medical Center - Crimson Care Collaborative, a student-faculty collaborative primary care practice. The didactic sessions underscore the importance of conducting an oral examination as an integral component of a primary care visit. Teaching-learning strategies include interprofessional faculty and students cofacilitating case discussions; problem-based cases designed to foster collaboration between dental, medical, nurse practitioner, and pharmacy students in the assessment, diagnosis, and treatment of older adult patients presenting with an oral-systemic condition or interaction; and dental students teaching health sciences students how to conduct an oral health examination and screening.

Leveraging educational technologies

Simulation-learning is an innovative approach to integrating oral health across health sciences curricula, and preparing primary care health professionals with the competencies to address oral health in every primary care visit and across a variety of primary care settings. The Arnold S. Goldstein Simulation Laboratories Suite at Bouvé College is dedicated to linking IPE and clinical practice. The Oral Health TIPS program leverages simulation-learning to create realistic representations of primary care practice environments through a variety of activities and technologies, ranging from low-technology role-playing to high-fidelity human patient simulators. Simulated environments may include community health centers, school-based programs, retail medical clinics, pharmacies, and other primary care settings. Simulation scenarios are designed to replicate real-life primary care clinical encounters. Health sciences students across Bouvé College engage with dental students from other academic institutions in team-based simulations focused on oral health promotion and oral disease prevention for healthy aging across the life cycle. The team-based simulations use standardized patients (trained actors) and debriefing techniques to enhance a patient-centered approach to integrating oral health as a component of comprehensive primary care.

Designing experiential learning

Innovations in experiential learning, such as cooperative education and community service, serve as a nexus between IPE and collaborative practice. Experiential learning provides students with real-life situations working with interprofessional teams in a community setting or practice environment, and the opportunity to apply concepts about oral health and healthy aging across the life cycle. A well-designed community service-learning experience is an effective strategy to increase student's awareness of oral health inequities and the underlying determinants of poor oral health for different population groups. For example, faculty and students from Bouvé College participated in a community service outreach to the Wampanoag Tribe of Gay Head (Aquinnah) on Martha's Vineyard, Massachusetts, led by Dr Brian Swann from Harvard School of Dental Medicine. Health sciences students collaborate with dental students and faculty in conducting oral health screenings, risk assessments, and health histories. Students interact in an interprofessional way with tribal community members by providing oral health information and counseling about healthy personal behaviors. Bringing together students and faculty across health professions in a community outreach is a promising approach to enhance interprofessional teamwork competencies, and promote the integration of oral health as an important component of general health.

INTERPROFESSIONAL COLLABORATIVE PRACTICE IN ACTION

...Very much like the model, should be national model of care, encourages cost effective care, makes smart financial decisions, includes the patient in the care plan...

—Joe Stanley

The US population is aging and the number of people living with chronic conditions grows to levels not ever seen before. The resulting burden on the system is already being felt: national long-term care spending in 2007 neared $207 billion, of which about 62% was spent on expenses related to nursing home care.[29] End-of-life health care costs continue to grow; by 2050, they are projected to be twice the current levels. To manage the inevitable strains on the health care system in the years to come, there will be an unprecedented need for multidisciplinary models of care to reduce cost and to raise system efficiency in the delivery of care. In particular, policy makers have started to focus on community- and home-based long-term care as a way to curb costs.[30] This section introduces and discusses one such multidisciplinary practice model, Program of All-inclusive Care for the Elderly (PACE), which has great promise in providing efficient and effective care. Over the years, PACE has grown from its quiet beginnings to become an integral part of modern home-based long-term care models.[31]

PACE is a nonprofit, multidisciplinary medical home program for the elderly funded by the federal government to provide eligible elderly a concierge-type patient-centered care. The PACE care model started in San Francisco, CA in the 1970s, when a Chinatown community decided to care for its elderly to avoid their unnecessary admission into nursing homes and hospitals.[32,33] A few years later, Dr William Gee, a dentist, together with the University of California San Francisco created the On-lok Senior Health Services, in which elderly receive all of their health care needs from the same place.[33] The original PACE care model offered these minimums: primary care services, social services, restorative therapies, personal care, nutrition, counseling, supportive care, and meal services.[32,34] It has grown to include additional services on-site including an oral health and dental clinic, planned daily activities, games, exercise, and personal and cosmetic care activities. There are presently 104 PACE programs in 31 states, and this number continues to grow.[35]

An important reason for the success of PACE is reduction in health care costs: with PACE the average monthly savings of using a community-based model of care versus nursing home admission is about $3632 per patient per month.[36,37] Equally important to its success, PACE allows the elderly to maintain their autonomy in decision making and to stay in their own homes for a longer amount of time, and the coordination of care through a "one-stop shop" model in which care providers work together to manage the patient's care. With respect to oral care, some PACE centers offer an on-site oral health clinic.[33] Most, however, contract with an independent dentist to work on-site. An on-site oral health clinic offers several benefits, such as lower dental care cost; improved accessibility to oral health care; regular continuous monitoring patients' oral health condition; and regular weekly updates of patients' medical, social, living, and medication changes. Unique to the Elder Service Plan of the North Shore's PACE program is the collaborative agreement with the Beth Israel Deaconess Medical Center's Interdisciplinary Geriatric Fellowship in Dental, Medical and Mental/Behavioral Health supported by the US Department of Health and Human Services, Health Resources and Services Administration. In the practice setting of Elder Service Plan of the North Shore, IPE is integrated into this model to improve health outcomes in the care and management of older adults and enrich medical/dental training. Working side by side in the same facility, the geriatric fellows learn from each other and practice collaborative and coordinated care aligned to the health care goals of each participant. There is a vital need for integrating oral health care into the elderly patients' overall treatment planning and management of care. Oral health care has seen great improvements in knowledge and clinical skill in the last century, during which there grew a developed body of literature that unequivocally linked poor oral health to overall health problems. For example, poor periodontal health and active disease in the oral cavity have been linked to systemic conditions, such as aspiration pneumonia (a leading cause of death in the elderly), diabetes, Alzheimer's disease, rapid weight loss, and cardiovascular condition.[38–46] All of these are examples of how oral health condition has an important effect on the patient's quality of life and longevity.

To better understand the benefit of the PACE model of care and how oral health can be integrated within it, we examine a common scenario encountered by a geriatric dentist. We present this case (**Box 3**) to highlight the breadth and comprehensiveness of care that a dentist is able to deliver to the geriatric patient.[47] The case also showcases the vital role a dentist can play in overall patient management and end-of-life planning involving one of the commonly diagnosed conditions in the elderly: Alzheimer's disease. The oral health care provider has a vital role from the beginning to the end in managing Alzheimer's patients.

The PACE model of care has been continuously growing.[48] Although each PACE site operates differently and independently, the guiding principle remains the same: combining a multidisciplinary approach with a patient-centered model. This model has provided a medium in which all health professionals work together in providing comprehensive care to the patients. The model allows for oral health care providers to interact directly with the primary care provider, patient's nurse, physical therapist, and counselor and to provide oral health services and treatment recommendations in

---

Box 3
The value of an interdisciplinary, patient-centered care model

Mr Smith is 75 years old and has recently enrolled into the PACE program. He was previously diagnosed with Alzheimer's disease, diabetes, hypertension, fibromyalgia, arthritis, and hyperlipidemia. He suffered a motor vehicle accident about 8 years ago, which damaged his lumbar spine. Since then, he has been living with chronic lower back pain. He can drive short distances but long distances are often hard on him. He lost his wife in this accident. His children have also moved away because of their employment conditions. He has a younger brother living with him, but the two do not have a good relationship. They decided to share a house because of Mr Smith's financial difficulties, so that he does not lose his house. Mr Smith has had considerable difficulty ever since his accident and his resulting inability to work—especially when his children moved away. During the cold season, he is often unable to leave the house for days because of pain. As his dementia advances, life is becoming more and more difficult for him. He and his children together decided to enroll him at the local PACE center.

Mr Smith married his high school sweetheart when he was 18. His wife worked at a fast food restaurant for many years and Mr Smith was a carpenter. They had two children who lived nearby until about 5 years ago. Mr Smith's only family is now his younger brother who works at a car shop. Mr Smith is extremely social and has many friends that continuously help him out, especially on days when he cannot leave his house. The only thing that bothers him is his continuous fights with his brother.

Today Mr Smith has come to the PACE center for his regular check-ups and to see the onsite dentist to start his oral health treatment. This is Mr Smith's second visit at PACE since his enrollment 3 weeks ago. So far he is extremely happy with the care and services that he has been receiving.

Geriatric dental assessment: oral, systemic, capability, autonomy, and reality
Oral Examination

Patient is edentulous and has been wearing dentures for 15 years. His current dentures set is his second. He does not recall what happened with his lower denture but reports to you that he cleans his dentures nightly. Your intraoral examination shows the following:

- Mr Smith's upper denture looks like this

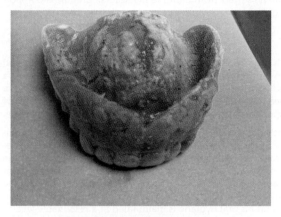

- When you elevate his upper lip you find this lesion

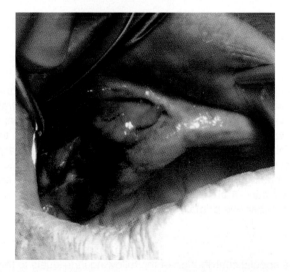

Systemic Examination

Alzheimer's disease, diabetes, hypertension, fibromyalgia, arthritis, and hyperlipidemia.

Capability

Patient reports that he is able to accomplish his personal care without any problems by himself. However, based on your assessment of his oral health condition, you realize that the patient's dentures are not cleaned daily. You observe denture stomatitis on the upper jaw along with gingival hyperplasia and denture sore suggestive that his dentures have not been removed from his mouth for a long time. His lower jaw was unremarkable, suggesting that the patient probably lost his lower dentures a long time ago.

Autonomy

The patient consents for his treatment, but his daughter and son, who live in another state, are also his health proxy.

Reality

The patient is the only person who is currently caring for himself. At the same time, he does require additional help. In addition, he suffers from multiple medical conditions, and importantly, he is dealing with advancing dementia.

Case summary

It is no secret that good oral health plays an important role in systemic health, and that good oral hygiene aids in the prevention of infectious diseases, such as aspiration pneumonia. As a patient's dementia progresses, oral hygiene and oral examinations in many cases become more challenging. Presenting the oral health care team from the beginning in the management of these patients is an important component of the multidisciplinary, patient-centered care team.

Mr Smith is a patient who is currently not working and is dealing with chronic pain and conditions that limit his ability to care for himself. He also suffers from a progressively advancing dementia, and his oral health needs daily care. Being part of an interdisciplinary team allows the dentist to start working with the patient at the first time that the dementia is diagnosed. Dentists are able to train the patient's caregiver and primary care team on how best to carry out the daily oral health routine for the patient. Being part of the PACE program, the dentist can regularly check the patient and ensure that his oral hygiene is maintained at a reasonable level.

consultation with other health care professionals. In this model, dentists and dental hygienists are an integrated part of the primary care team.

SUMMARY

Advancing oral health necessitates new models of IPE and practice that are responsive to the complex oral and systemic health needs of an aging society. The Oral Health TIPS program is an innovative IPE model that aims to prepare the next generation of health professionals with oral health and team-based competencies to strengthen the primary care health system and integrate oral health in every primary care visit. This innovative model holds great promise for linking IPE and clinical practice through innovations in technology, instruction, and experiential learning. The PACE model of patient-centered care is an exemplar for integrating oral health as an essential component of comprehensive primary care.

ACKNOWLEDGMENTS

The authors acknowledge the special contribution of the following individuals to the development and implementation of the Innovations in Interprofessional Oral Health program: Pamela Ring, JD, MPA, Ashwini Ranade, BDS, MPH, and Kathryn Robinson, BSN, MHA/Ed, Northeastern University; Kerry Maguire, DDS, MSPH, The Forsyth Institute; Romesh Nalliah, BDS, and Brian Swann, DDS, MPH, Harvard School of Dental Medicine; Amy Weinstein, MD, MPH, Beth Israel Deaconess Medical Center - Crimson Care Collaborative; Ellen Patterson, MD, MA, and Dorothy Vannah, MEd, RDH, Tufts University School of Dental Medicine; and Wendy Gammon, MA, MEd, University of Massachusetts Medical School. They also thank numerous faculty and students from Bouvé College of Health Sciences, Northeastern University who participated in the first-year implementation of this program and who provided invaluable feedback for improving program effectiveness. Special thanks to Mr Joe Stanley, site manager at PACE community in Lynn, MA, who has contributed important insights into patient-centered care and interdisciplinary practice. Ashwini Ranade assisted with technical preparation of this article.

REFERENCES

1. Flexner A. Medical education in the United States and Canada: a report to the Carnegie Foundation for the advancement of teaching. New York: The Carnegie Foundation for the Advancement of Teaching; 1910. Available at: http://www.carnegiefoundation.org/sites/default/files/elibrary/Carnegie_Flexner_Report.pdf.
2. Welch WH, Rose W. Institute of hygiene: a report to the General Education Board of Rockefeller Foundation. New York: The Rockefeller Foundation; 1915.
3. The Committee for the Study of Nursing Education. Nursing and nursing education in the United States. New York: The Rockefeller Foundation; 1923.
4. Gies WJ, Pritchett H. Dental education in the United States and Canada: a report to the Carnegie Foundation for the advancement of teaching. New York: The Carnegie Foundation for the Advancement of Teaching; 1926.
5. Frenk J, Chen L, Bhutta ZA, et al. Health professionals for a new century: transforming education to strengthen health systems in an interdependent world. Lancet 2010;376(9756):1923–58. Available at: http://dash.harvard.edu/bitstream/handle/1/4626403/Ed_HealthProfCommisionp5_40.PDF?sequence=1.
6. Beaglehole R, Benzian H, Crail J, et al. Oral health atlas: mapping a neglected global health issue. Cointrin (Switzerland): 2009. Available at: http://issuu.com/myriadeditions/docs/flipbook_oral_health. Accessed December 31, 2013.
7. Population ageing and development: ten years after Madrid. 2012. Available at: http://www.un.org/en/development/desa/population/publications/pdf/popfacts/popfacts_2012-4.pdf. Accessed December 31, 2013.
8. United States Department of Health and Human Services, Office of the Surgeon General. Oral Health in America: a report of the Surgeon General. Rockville (MD): National Institute of Dental and Craniofacial Research, National Institutes of Health; 2000. Available at: http://www.surgeongeneral.gov/library/reports/oralhealth/index.html.
9. Institute of Medicine. Improving access to oral health care for vulnerable and underserved populations. Washington, DC: Institute of Medicine; 2011. Available at: http://www.iom.edu/reports/2011/improving-access-to-oral-health-care-for-vulnerable-and-underserved-populations.aspx.
10. Institute of Medicine. Advancing oral health in America. Washington, DC: Institute of Medicine; 2011. Available at: http://www.iom.edu/Reports/2011/Advancing-Oral-Health-in-America.aspx.
11. United States Department of Health and Human Services. National call to action to promote oral health. Rockville (MD): US Department of Health and Human Services, Public Health Service, National Institutes of Health, National Institute of Dental and Craniofacial Research; 2003. Available at: http://www.surgeongeneral.gov/library/calls/oralhealth/nationalcalltoaction.html.
12. Schmitt MH, Gilbert JHV, Brandt BF, et al. The coming of age for interprofessional education and practice. Am J Med 2013;126:284–8. Available at: http://www.ncbi.nlm.nih.gov/pubmed/23415053.
13. World Health Organization Study Group on Interprofessional Education and Collaborative Practice. Framework for action on interprofessional education and

collaborative practice. Geneva (Switzerland): World Health Organization; 2010. Available at: http://whqlibdoc.who.int/hq/2010/WHO_HRH_HPN_10.3_eng.pdf.

14. Interprofessional Education Collaborative Expert Panel. Core competencies for interprofessional collaborative practice: a report of an expert panel. Washington, DC: Interprofessional Education Collaborative; 2011. Available at: http://www.aacn.nche.edu/education-resources/ipecreport.pdf.

15. Institute of Medicine. Educating for the health team. Washington, DC: Institute of Medicine; 1972.

16. Institute of Medicine. Executive summary: health professions education: a bridge to quality. Washington, DC: Institute of Medicine; 2003. Available at: http://www.iom.edu/Reports/2003/health-professions-education-a-bridge-to-quality.aspx.

17. Global forum on innovations in health professional education. Available at: http://www.iom.edu/Activities/Global/InnovationHealthProfEducation.aspx. Accessed December 31, 2013.

18. Westphal CM, Furnari W, Haber J. College of Dentistry/College of Nursing partnership. Access 2009;23(6):18, 21.

19. Alfano M. Connecting dental education to other health professions. J Dent Educ 2012;76(1):46–50.

20. Haber J, Strasser S, Lloyd M, et al. The oral-systemic connection in primary care. Nurse Pract 2009;34(3):43–8.

21. Djukic M, Fulmer T, Adams JG, et al. NYU3T: teaching, technology, teamwork. A model for interprofessional education scalability and sustainability. Nurs Clin North Am 2012;47:333–46.

22. Geriatric interdisciplinary team training (GITT) program. 2011. Available at: http://hartfordign.org/education/gitt/. Accessed December 13, 2013.

23. TeamSTEPPS. 2013. Available at: http://teamstepps.ahrq.gov. Accessed December 13, 2013.

24. Dolce MC, Haber J, Shelley D, et al. Oral health nursing education and practice program. Nurs Res Pract 2012;2012:149673. http://dx.doi.org/10.1155/2012/149673.

25. Fulmer T, Cabrera P. The primary care visit? What else could be happening? Nurs Res Pract 2012;2012:720506. http://dx.doi.org/10.1155/2012/720506.

26. National Interprofessional Initiative on Oral Health. Clinicians for oral health. 2011. Available at: http://www.niioh.org. Accessed December 16, 2013.

27. Clark MB, Douglass AB, Maier R, et al. Smiles for life: a national oral health curriculum. 3rd edition. 2010. Available at: http://elearning.talariainc.com/buildcontent.aspx?tut=555&pagekey=62948&cbreceipt=0. Accessed December 19, 2013.

28. Dolce M. Nurse faculty enrichment and competency development in oral-systemic health. Nurs Res Pract 2012;2012:567058. http://dx.doi.org/10.1155/2012/567058.

29. Komisar HL, Shirey L. National spending for long-term care. Washington, DC: Health Policy Institute, Georgetown University; 2007.

30. Long-term care: issues and policy considerations. Available at: http://www.mffh.org/mm/files/FactSheetLTC.pdf. Accessed December 19, 2013.

31. Eng C, Pedulla J, Eleazer GP, et al. Program of All-inclusive Care for the Elderly (PACE): an innovative model of integrated geriatric care and financing. J Am Geriatr Soc 1997;45(2):223–32.

32. Lee W, Eng C, Fox N, et al. PACE: a model for integrated care of frail older patients. Program of All-inclusive Care for the Elderly. Geriatrics 1998;53(6):65–9.

33. PACE innovation act reaches milestone. 2013. Available at: http://www.npaonline.org. Accessed December 19, 2013.

34. United States Department of Health and Human Services, Centers for Medicare and Medicaid Services. Quick facts about Programs of All-inclusive Care for the Elderly (PACE). Washington, DC: Centers for Medicare and Medicaid; 2011. Available at: http://www.medicare.gov/Pubs/pdf/11341.pdf. Accessed July 25, 2014.

35. National PACE Association. Who, what, and where is PACE? Alexandria, VA: National PACE Association; 2014. Available at: http://www.npaonline.org/website/article.asp?id=12&title=Who,_What_and_Where_Is_PACE? Accessed July 25, 2014.

36. Hirth V, Baskins J, Dever-Bumba M. Program of All-inclusive Care (PACE): past, present, and future. J Am Med Dir Assoc 2009;10(3):155–60. Available at: http://www.dhcs.ca.gov/provgovpart/Documents/Waiver Renewal/PACE_Article_JAMDA_091.pdf.

37. Costs of care. Available at: http://longtermcare.gov/costs-how-to-pay/costs-of-care/. Accessed December 19, 2013.

38. Newman MG, Takei H, Perry R, et al. Carranza's clinical periodontology. 10th edition. Philadelphia, PA: Saunders Elsevier; 2006.

39. Stein P, Steffen M, Smith C, et al. Serum antibodies to periodontal pathogens are a risk factor for Alzheimer's disease. Alzheimers Dement 2012;8:196–203.

40. Stein PS, Desrosiers M, Donegan SJ, et al. Tooth loss, dementia and neuropathology in the Nun Study. J Am Dent Assoc 2007;138:1314–22.

41. Steward R. Mouths and brains. Could oral infection be a risk factor for dementia? J Neurol Neurosurg Psychiatry 2009;80:1184.

42. Sarin J, Balasubramaniam R, Corcoran AM, et al. Reducing the risk of aspiration pneumonia among elderly patients in long-term care facilities through oral health interventions. J Am Med Dir Assoc 2008;9(2):128–35.

43. Moodley A, Wood NH, Shangase S. The relationship between periodontitis and diabetes: a brief review. SADJ 2013;68(6):260–4.

44. Shangase SL, Mohangi GU, Hassam-Essa S, et al. The association between periodontitis and systemic health: an overview. SADJ 2013;68(1):8, 10–12.

45. Suzuki K, Nomura T, Sakurai M, et al. Relationship between number of present teeth and nutritional intake in institutionalized elderly. Bull Tokyo Dent Coll 2005;46(4):135–43. Available at: http://ir.tdc.ac.jp/irucaa/bitstream/10130/242/1/46_135.pdf.

46. Syrjälä AM, Pussinen PI, Komulainen K, et al. Salivary flow rate and risk of malnutrition: a study among dentate, community-dwelling older people. Gerodontology 2013;30(4):270–5.

47. Laudenbach JM, Jacobsen PL, Mohammad AR, et al. Clinician's guide oral health in geriatric patients. 3rd edition. Edmonds, WA: American Academy of Oral Medicine; 2010.

48. Turk L, Parmley J, Ames A, et al. A new era in home care. Semin Nurse Manag 2000;8(3):143–50.

Innovations in Dental Care Delivery for the Older Adult

Lynn Ann Bethel, RDH, MPH[a],*, Esther E. Kim, DMD, MPH[b], Charles M. Seitz, DDS, MPH[c,d], Brian J. Swann, DDS, MPH[c,e]

KEYWORDS

- Public health • Workforce • Innovative • Access • Older adults

KEY POINTS

- Access to and reducing disparities in oral health for older adults is a complex problem that requires innovative strategies. Offering oral health care services in alternative settings, such as senior centers, places that are familiar to older adults, and where physical limitations can be better accommodated, is a key strategy to increase access and reduce disparities.
- The success of the strategy of oral health care in alternative settings necessitates supporting the utilization of dental hygienists in public health settings including long-term care facilities, creating new dental providers, as well as to a collaborative practice approach whereby both dental and nondental professionals coordinate care.
- It is incumbent on the dental professional to take the next steps by: (1) promoting the incorporation of the oral health needs of seniors in dental and dental hygiene education, in addition to continuing education courses; (2) training medical and other nondental professionals serving seniors on how to perform oral health assessments and promote collaborative care between the professions; and (3) supporting the development of new health policies that prioritize oral health for older adults as a primary health care agenda.

INTRODUCTION

The new cohort of seniors, those born between 1946 and 1964, are different from the older cohorts in that they are more likely to retain their dentition, placing them at a

No financial disclosures or conflicts of interest.
[a] Commonwealth of Massachusetts, 3270 Covent Garden Drive, Reno, NV 89509, USA; [b] New York State Department of Health, Bureau of Dental Health, Room 957, ESP Corning Tower, Albany, NY 12237, USA; [c] Harvard School of Dental Medicine, 188 Longwood Avenue, Boston, MA 02115, USA; [d] 1047 Belmont Street, Watertown, MA 02472, USA; [e] Oral Health Department, Cambridge Health Alliance Windsor Street Health Center, 119 Windsor Street, Cambridge, MA 02139, USA
* Corresponding author.
E-mail address: LynnABethel@aol.com

http://dx.doi.org/10.1016/j.cden.2014.07.003
0011-8532/14/$ – see front matter © 2014 Elsevier Inc. All rights reserved.
dental.theclinics.com

higher risk for oral diseases.[1] However, older adults frequently do not access oral health care. According to the 1996 and 2004 Medical Expenditure Panel Survey, only 46% of older adults aged 65 to 74 and 39% of older adults aged 75 and older reported visiting a dentist.[2]

Multiple factors contribute to low and limited access to dental care, including the supply and distribution of experienced dental professionals. Limited infrastructure particularly, in rural areas of the country, and the supply of dental professionals with the required training needed to provide for the particular needs of older adults[3,4] play a key role, in addition to the limited interaction between dental professionals and other health professionals who regularly care for this high-risk population.

DENTAL AND DENTAL HYGIENE EDUCATION

The number and distribution of dentists and dental hygienists within the population is an important factor in assessing how well the dental profession is meeting the current needs of the public, especially those 65 years and older, the fastest growing segment of the American population. Excluding the District of Columbia, the dentists to population ratio by state ranged from 31.3 to 69 per 100,000 residents.[5] In the United States, there are more than 190,000 licensed dental hygienists,[6] an average ratio of 50 dental hygienists per 100,000 population.[7]

Owing to the number of experienced dentists retiring or dying, the number of new dental professionals entering the profession is just as important. In 2013 there were 66 accredited dental schools in the United States and 10 in Canada. Each year there are approximately 21,000 students enrolled in predoctoral education programs, and recent trends demonstrate an increase in dental school enrollment similar to that of the early 1980s. In 2010 there were about 4800 dental school graduates or a ratio of about 1 graduating dentist for every 64,000 Americans; and although many choose to practice within a specialty, few choose geriatrics.[8] There are 332 dental hygiene schools in the United States, and annually, more than 6700 graduate from entry-level programs receiving an Associate's or Bachelor's degree.[9] By 2020, it is expected that 44% more dental hygienists than dentists will graduate annually.[10]

THE PRACTICE OF DENTISTRY: IS THERE A NEED TO CHANGE?

While medicine has gradually shifted away from solo practice, leading to expanded skill levels and specialization within professions, an increased allied health care workforce, and the addition of new technicians and other assistants,[11,12] this same shift has been slow in dentistry. Dentists primarily continue to work in small solo and group private practices, and the role and scope of practice of dental providers remain fairly static and well defined.[11,12] In recent years, this traditional provision of dental care has been scrutinized, particularly in its inadequacy to meet the increasing oral health needs of older adults.

Long-term concern may be warranted for the 10,000 Americans retiring daily, as it is estimated that only 2% of the baby-boomers turning age 65 will have access to dental insurance benefits[13] and admission to the traditional dental delivery system. For some older adults, dental care is being accessed through emergency rooms, a result of a shrinking workforce. Emergency room visits that were dental-related among adults older than 65 years rose from 1 million from 1999/2000 to 2.3 million during 2009/2010.[14] Others access care through Federally Qualified Health Centers (FQHC), which provide comprehensive oral health care services to low-income and uninsured individuals in underserved communities.[15] At the national level, the number of these FQHCs has increased 58% from 1997 to 2004,[16] and totaled 1128 in 2011.[16] With 31 states

(62%) having high rates of dental Health Provider Shortage Areas (HPSAs) and meeting only 40% or less of dental provider needs,[15] it is essential that alternative strategies for the delivery of dental care are implemented. This approach includes providing care in nondental settings such as senior centers, nursing homes, and long-term care facilities, and in the home. By expanding access to dental care into existing community venues that are already regularly frequented by the target population, key factors such as transportation costs, patient anxiety, and empty appointment slots, to name a few, are either reduced or eliminated.[17]

Infrastructure and workforce barriers limit older adults from obtaining appropriate care, driving health care costs higher and the quality of life lower. The need for better oral health care for the seniors is readily apparent. Against this backdrop, these issues may be addressed through innovative models and policies focused on the delivery of oral health care. Increasing access to oral health care for older adults is a complex problem that requires creative solutions. A key strategy that addresses this problem is to alter the traditional provision of dental services by creating new environments that facilitate easy access.[17]

NEW TRENDS IN DENTAL EDUCATION AND PRACTICE

In most dental programs, predoctoral dental students are trained in medicine for as long as 2 years; however, once they matriculate their medical knowledge is underused. An encouraging step in the renaissance in dental education is to allow dentists to be trained at the capacity of a mid-level medical provider. Today, a dental resident who is doing a rotation in internal medicine is required to function at the level of a third-year medical student (conducting patient interviews, doing basic medical examinations, and making referrals); thus a dentist is a de facto oral physician (OP).

The Cambridge Health Alliance (CHA) Windsor Street Health Center (WSHC) is actively implementing a training model known as the OP.[18] The CHA is a large safety-net organization with 3 hospitals and 12 clinic sites west of Boston, Massachusetts, with its catchment area consisting of approximately 400,000 residents. Within the Oral Health Department, more than 90% of patients seen receive public health dental benefits. A General Practice Residency program, affiliated with the Harvard School of Dental Medicine, exposes recent graduates to a 1-year general dentistry program with an emphasis on public health.

If medicine, in a limited capacity, were incorporated into a dental practice it could have an impact on primary care to strengthen best overall health practices. In addition to conducting the medical interview, the OP takes blood pressure, oxygen level, height and weight to measure body mass index, and dental radiographs, and conducts extraoral and intraoral examinations. With this information, the provider discusses the findings and makes recommendations for treatment. Blood tests and/or urine tests can also be ordered if they are in the best interest of the patient. Often this decision is driven by the lack of access to a primary care physician (PCP). Most importantly, the OP can expedite the recommendation for patients to see their PCP for follow-up care or can directly contact that PCP to discuss the best approaches to treatment. These encounters develop rapport, and cross-training stimulates interprofessional learning for the benefit of the patient. Reinforcing the application of medical knowledge and demonstrating the relationship between mental health, oral health, and systemic health in everyday clinical care is ongoing. Surveys are being developed to ascertain whether patients are comfortable with an OP (dentist) asking in-depth health questions as part of the medical interview.

Additional benefits of this model include an increased knowledge to dental providers of how medications interact with oral health treatment, and improved communications with physicians and allied health professionals. By educating physicians and nurses at grand-round presentations, CHA is not only raising oral-systemic health knowledge, it is also bridging the gap between medicine and dentistry, and thus revising and complementing the interdisciplinary patient-centered health care model.

In addition to the interdisciplinary efforts, a more effective patient history and physical workup model has been implemented using patient interview techniques, such as in studies by Rosenthal and Rosnow.[19] These studies demonstrated that a face-to-face medical interview is significantly more reliable than the written questionnaire. For example, when treating older adults it is not uncommon for clinicians to encounter problems with incomplete or inaccurate medical forms. The stimulation provided by the open dialogue leads to better recall about the patient's health history. The OP validates the patient as an individual by spending more time conducting the medical interview and demonstrating a caring attitude, promoting the first stage of "healing." The knowledge gained potentially increases health literacy for both patients and providers. This increase has a positive impact on health care outcomes and costs.

COLLABORATIVE PRACTICE AMONG DENTAL PROVIDERS

The success in altering the traditional provision of dental services may be linked to collaborative practice arrangements among both dental providers and nondental professionals. This approach also entails expanding the scope of practice of both dental and nondental providers, and creating new types of dental providers altogether. In particular, the dental auxiliary personnel, including the dental hygienist and the dental therapist, can play a pivotal role in increasing access to oral health care for older adults.

Collaborative practice is a health care workforce innovation designed to coordinate care among providers, and its use in dentistry is a form of practice that is only just taking shape. Collaborative practice in a dental setting involves the dental auxiliary personnel, usually a dental hygienist or a dental therapist, and the dentist. Although several states have currently arranged some form of collaborative practice, there is no single model. Across several states, a collaborative practice between the dental auxiliary personnel and the dentist can differ in its level of agreement between the providers, the extent of supervision the dentist provides, special education and/or experience requirements for the dental auxiliary personnel, and types of services that the dental auxiliary personnel can provide to specific types of populations (**Box 1**).[20]

Furthermore, collaborative practice arrangements among providers can increase the effectiveness of providing care in nondental settings. In essence, the various legislation, regulations, and training allow the dental auxiliary personnel to provide care

---

Box 1
Direct-access states

Direct access means that the dental hygienist can initiate treatment based on his or her assessment of patients' needs without the specific authorization of a dentist, treat patients without the presence of a dentist, and maintain a provider-patient relationship.

Alaska	Arizona	Arkansas	California	Colorado	Connecticut
Florida	Idaho	Iowa	Kansas	Kentucky	Maine
Massachusetts	Michigan	Minnesota	Missouri	Montana	Nebraska
New Hampshire	New Mexico	New York	Nevada	Ohio	Oklahoma
Oregon	Pennsylvania	Rhode Island	South Carolina	South Dakota	Tennessee
Texas	Vermont	Virginia	Washington	West Virginia	Wisconsin

From American Dental Hygienists' Association. Available at: http://www.adha.org/direct-access. Accessed December 15, 2013.

outside of traditional dental offices.[17] For example, a dental hygienist can be either certified or receive a "public health endorsement" to offer some level of preventive care in public health or nondental settings without the supervision of a dentist.[17] The dental auxiliary personnel could further coordinate care with caregivers, including nursing staff and aides, to deliver preventive services. In 2013 there were 36 "direct-access" states, meaning that the dental hygienist can initiate treatment based on his or her assessment of patient's needs without the specific authorization of a dentist, treat the patient without the presence of a dentist, and maintain a provider-patient relationship.[20]

Specifically, public health dental hygienist (PHDH) is a collaborative practice between the dental hygienist and the dentist.[21] Enabled by legislation, a dental hygienist can enter into an agreement approved by the state board of dental examiners with a licensed dentist that designates authorization for the services provided by the dental hygienist. The PHDH is allowed to access different segments of the underserved and vulnerable populations in nondental settings, such as schools, institutions, nursing and public health facilities, and group homes.[20,21] In many states, the PHDH is directly responsible for finding a referring dentist who will provide the necessary treatment for patients who have received preventive care. In addition, they may also be directly reimbursed by the patient, Medicaid, or private insurance (although this varies by state). In 2013, 15 state Medicaid programs had regulations that supported direct reimbursement to a dental hygienist.[22]

In Massachusetts, the PHDH was enabled by legislation in 2009 with the purpose of increasing access to dental care for high-risk populations, including older adults. However, in an informal interview in 2013, 2 years after the legislation was implemented, it was revealed that while a few PHDHs did provide services for older adults in nursing homes and long-term care facilities, many predominantly provided services to children, citing among other reasons that it was challenging to coordinate care with caregivers who do not perceive oral health as important.[23] More structural changes, such as placing a higher priority on oral health in institutional, care are needed to help maximize the utilization of dental hygienists in these alternative settings.

The dental therapist, advanced dental hygiene practitioner, and community dental health coordinator are new members of the dental team whose utilization in nondental settings, especially senior centers, nursing homes, and long-term care facilities, should be further explored.[24,25] Alaska and Minnesota currently use dental therapists, whose services range from preventive and some restorative care to treatment planning and nonsurgical extractions of permanent teeth.[21] Their wider scope of practice can be particularly useful for high-risk older adults, such as those who are institutionalized or homebound.

To have better health outcomes and create a "true" medical home, solutions must address cost containment, improve accessibility, reduce barriers, and raise oral health literacy.

CROSS-TRAINING AND COLLABORATIVE CARE

Cross-talk and cross-training are essential to an interdisciplinary, collaborative approach that can provide comprehensive patient care. Significant evidence exists supporting the effectiveness of cross-training between dental professionals and other medical and health professions such as physicians, nurse practitioners, physician assistants, nurses, nutritionists, and social workers.

Through this collaborative approach, oral health care can be better integrated into primary health care, which has more routine contact with high-risk populations, including seniors. On average seniors see their primary health care provider about 5.5 times annually,[26] providing more opportunities for preliminary dental and oral screenings and education, in addition to the incorporation of clinical services into primary care medicine.[27] For instance, monitoring the oral health of older adults could be integrated into a chronic care model and be offered in systemic primary care carried out by family physicians. This approach can especially benefit, for example, Medicare recipients with no dental coverage or a senior living with a chronic disease such as diabetes.

In addition, the role of nonhealth professionals, such as social workers, should be further explored, as they can play an essential role in helping older adults connect to oral health systems. As social workers have been working with medical professionals since the early 1990s, they too can be a significant partner of the dental professional[28]; they represent an ideal partner, as they already have the capacity to obtain the connections and partnerships with community agencies.[28]

An example of this collaborative approach to training and providing health care is the Geriatric Training Program for Physicians, Dentists, and Behavior and Mental Health Professionals supported by the Health Resource Services Administration. This grant supports the interprofessional training of Geriatric Medicine, Geriatric Dental, and Geriatric Behavior and Mental Health professionals in geriatrics. Specifically, The Harvard Geriatric Dental Fellowship program participates in cross-training with Beth Israel Deaconess Medical and Psychiatric Fellows through seminars on aging, the exposure to a multitude of different services and programs tailored to various populations of aging adults, and overlapping clinical experiences, specifically, monthly case conferences that discuss the status of the shared patient panel of a fellow from each discipline.

CREATIVE DENTAL DELIVERY SYSTEMS
The Group Denture Appointment

Innovation in the delivery of dental care should be addressed within this era of health care crisis. An approach to tackle the long waiting lists and the high costs associated with caring for denture patients is the "group visit." The group visit model is poised to encourage more private dental practices to consider treating patients with public health insurance by addressing historical barriers, including high no-show rates and low profit margins.

All individuals seen at the clinic are given the option of either a group visit or an individual appointment. In the group visit, 8 to 12 patients are treated at one time in a large conference room, not in the traditional office setting. Once it is determined that the person has chosen the group visit, he or she signs a consent form and receives an appointment every 2 weeks until the delivery of dentures. In the group visit model, up to 3 patients are seated in the front of the room facing away from the audience or other patients in the room; this is where treatment and measurements are made. The other patients in the room can only observe the dentist, and while waiting are able to read oral health material and/or listen to a presentation relative to their overall health and nutrition.

The concept of group visits was practiced by a psychologist, Edward Noffsinger, and a physician, J.C. Scott, from Kaiser Permanente Medical Center (Santa Clara, CA).[29] This appointment model was proposed for patients suffering from chronic illnesses such as diabetes and asthma. It was also seen as a way to improve access for more patients and to decrease waiting lists without increasing physician hours. In addition, the group visit scheme ameliorates the effects of late cancellations and no-shows. Under this model, patient satisfaction is positive, patient anxiety is lower, patients are able to learn from each other, and practice growth is evident.[30] Peer learning reinforces and comforts the patients who have been traumatized by dental pain and previous negative experiences. The size of the work space allows family, friends, and/or caregivers to accompany the patient, providing them support. In addition, nutritional training sessions are sometimes incorporated simultaneously while the denture model is in full operation.

To demonstrate the cost and time savings from the group denture visit, an analysis was conducted. The public health insurance benefit in Massachusetts to replace missing teeth is $680 per arch, which is slightly more than half the cost of $1200 per arch in the private sector. With one dentist and supporting staff, an average of 10 patients are seen within a 1.5-hour time slot when compared with seeing those same 10 patients in an individual model totaling 5 hours of chair time. The group denture patient can be scheduled every 2 weeks as opposed to the monthly, individual appointment. This consolidation of patients translates into reduced overheads. The profit margin for an individual appointment is $155 per arch. Because 3 patients can be seen within the same 30-minute time period (10 minutes per patient), the profit is $824 for the same 30-minute time period.

Placing Theory into Practice

A stagnant economy, the loss of spending power within the middle class, the Affordable Care Act, and an aging baby-boomer population who are in need of a wide range of dental services from prevention to rehabilitation has caused a rethink of how dental care should be delivered. In addition, dentistry seems to be entering a new era with the dental economy remaining flat,[30] providing the general dentist an opportunity to rethink where, how, and to whom she or he may provide care as time goes by.

One model, implemented for more than 30 years by Charles M. Seitz, incorporates into his 2-chair, 3.5-day per week general practice located outside Boston, Massachusetts, a subpractice that serves seniors living in 17 long-term care facilities within the catchment area of his practice. To implement his subpractice, Dr Seitz collaborates with 5 PHDHs all working part-time. He also has access to a wheelchair-accessible dental clinic located nearby. The subpractice model limits missed appointments and lost revenue.

The advantage of this public health subpractice lies in the simplicity of the equipment used, costing about $800, and the ease of administration in that all billing is processed through the main dental practice. By having a "nursing home kit" ready, a dentist can easily go to a local long-term care facility (LTCF) where there are patients who need care (**Box 2**).

In the LTCF, the dentist's duties include performing examinations and oral cancer screenings, treatment planning, providing sedative restorations using glass ionomer cement, and denture fabrication and adjustments; no hard- or soft-tissue manipulation is performed in the nursing facility setting. The patients who need more extensive procedures are transported to the wheelchair-accessible clinic routine operative and surgical care is performed. This approach allows close alignment with the health care team at the nursing facility while treating the medically compromised senior patient, delivering to health care providers immediate feedback on the treatment and follow-up care needed by the senior residents in their care. All instruments and materials are transported, disposed of, and/or sterilized at the primary dental office following state rules and regulations for the practice of dentistry.

Dr Seitz's dental care is offered in collaboration with PHDHs, licensed dental hygienists who provide preventive care within a public health setting such as the

---

Box 2
Items to be included in the "nursing home" kit

- Stanley Mobile Work Center (Stanley Tools US, New Britain, CT)
- Light-emitting diode headlamp (available at camping stores)
- Germicidal wipes
- Disposable mouth mirrors
- Scissors
- Vaseline
- Pulp tester
- Alginate, mixing bowl, spatula, impression trays
- Vinyl polysiloxane impression syringe gun, light body, medium body, blue mouse (3M ESPE Dental Products, St Paul, MN)
- Candle wax and electric heater for adjustment of bite rims (available at craft stores)
- Aseptico motor model AEU-03 for denture adjustments and prophylaxis (Aseptico, Inc, Woodinville, WA)
- Rope wax/pink base plate wax
- Prophy cups/paste
- Extension cord
- Instrument cassette
- Buffalo knife
- Glass ionomer cement, mixing pad, and spatula
- Enlarged, laminated copy of dental license

LTCF, without the supervision of a dentist. The PHDHs schedule their own appointments with the residents living in the LTCF, providing prophylaxis, topical fluoride applications, and digital radiographs, and uploading the images using cloud-based software for the dentist's diagnosis. The PHDHs also provide oral hygiene instruction to patients and in-service oral health education to facility personnel. All costs associated with the PHDH services are absorbed by the dental hygienists, who directly receive reimbursement from Medicaid and other sources for the services they provide.

Dr Seitz provides the restorative and rehabilitative dental care needed by the seniors, or the PHDHs make direct referrals to other licensed dentists based on their needs and/or the families' request. Utilizing dental hygienists who are allowed through state regulation to practice without a dentist on-site not only provides cost-effective preventive dental care but also provides for a referral source, expanding the use of dental services within the practice and increasing its revenue.

Dentists working in LTCFs are also in a position to collaborate with local dental and dental hygiene schools. All accredited dental and dental hygiene education programs include community-based rotations and, although each school may vary in its approach to public health dentistry, all are valuable resources within their community, especially to seniors. Harvard University School of Dental Medicine partners with Dr Seitz to provide predoctoral students and postdoctoral fellows lectures focused on treating geriatric patients, in addition to observational experiences at the facilities he serves. This approach provides the students and fellows valuable real-world exposure to the needs and limitations of the seniors living in long-term care. The students are also taught how to integrate dental treatment plans with medical treatment plans by working with physicians and nurse practitioners at the facilities, promoting integrated care. Most importantly, the students learn that the delivery of dental care does not necessarily need to occur in the traditional dental setting; potentially expanding access to care for seniors with limited mobility and/or living in other settings, including the housebound.

SUMMARY

As the United States population grows older and living with multiple chronic conditions becomes the new normal, unprecedented demands on the health care system will be made. To supply the resources to meet these demands, new paradigms of care are needed. Access to and reducing disparities in oral health for older adults is a complex problem that requires innovative strategies. Offering oral health care services in alternative settings, such as senior centers, places that are familiar to older adults, and where physical limitations can be better accommodated, is a key strategy to increase access and reduce disparities.[31–33] The success of this strategy may be linked to a collaborative practice approach whereby both dental and nondental professionals coordinate care. It is incumbent on the dental professional to take the next steps by: (1) promoting the incorporation of the oral health needs of seniors in dental and dental hygiene education, in addition to continuing education courses; (2) training medical and other nondental professionals serving seniors on how to perform oral health assessments and promote collaborative care between the professions; (3) supporting the utilization of dental hygienists in public health settings including LTCFs, and creating new dental providers; and (4) supporting the development of new health policies that prioritize oral health for older adults as a primary health care agenda.

REFERENCES

1. Institute of Medicine. The second fifty years: promoting health and preventing disability. Washington, DC: National Academy Press; 1992.
2. Manski RJ, Brown E. Dental use, expenses, private dental coverage, and changes, 1996 and 2004. Rockville (MD): Agency for Healthcare Research and Quality; 2007. MEPS Chartbook No.17.
3. Institute of Medicine and National Research Council. Improving access to oral health care for vulnerable and underserved populations. Washington, DC: The National Academies Press; 2011.
4. Vargas CM, Kramarrow EA, Yellowitz JA. The oral health of older Americans. Aging trends; No. 3. Hyattsville (MD): National Center for Health Statistics; 2001.
5. National Institute of Dental and Craniofacial Research. Oral health, U.S. 2002 annual report: Dental Care Workforce. 2002. Available at: http://drc.hhs.gov/report/16_5.htm. Accessed November 9, 2013.
6. Bureau of Labor and Statistics. Occupational employment and wages, May 2012: dental hygienists. Washington, DC: US Department of Labor; 2013. Available at: http://www.bls.gov/oes/current/oes292021.htm.
7. Center for Health Workforce Studies. A profile of active dental hygienists in New York. Albany (NY): School of Public Health University of Albany; 2011. Available at: www.health.ny.gov/health_care/medicaid/redesign/docs/profile_active_dental_hygienists_in_ny.pdf.
8. American Dental Educators' Association. Dentists and demographics: a Dean's briefing. 2013. Available at: www.adea.org/.../finalreviseddeans/dentistsdemographics.pdf. Accessed November 9, 2013.

9. American Dental Hygienists' Association. Facts about the Dental Hygiene Workforce in the United States. 2013. Available at: http://www.adha.org/resources-docs/75118_Facts_About_the_Dental_Hygiene_Workforce.pdf. Accessed November 13, 2013.

10. Solomon ES. The past and future evolution of the dental workforce team. J Dent Educ 2012;76(8):1028–35. Available at: http://www.jdentaled.org/content/76/8/1028.full.pdf+html.

11. Center for the Health Professions at the University of San Francisco, California. Collaborative practice in American dentistry: practice and potential. 2011. Available at: http://futurehealth.ucsf.edu/Content/29/2011-01_Collaborative_Practice_in_American_Dentistry_Practice_and_Potential.pdf. Accessed November 28, 2013.

12. Mertz E, O'Neil E. The growing challenge of providing oral health care services to all Americans. Health Aff (Millwood) 2002;21(5):65–77.

13. Department of Health and Human Services. Oral health in America: a report of the surgeon general. Rockville (MD): U.S. Department of Health and Human Services National Institute of Dental and Craniofacial Research, National Institute of Health; 2002.

14. National Hospital Ambulatory Care Survey. Available at: http://www.cdc.gov/nchs/ahcd.htm. Accessed December 1, 2013.

15. Oral Health America, State of Decay. Are older Americans coming of age without oral healthcare? Chicago: 2013. Available at: http://s.bsd.net/teeth/default/page/-/SODUpdate10.15.pdf. Accessed December 1, 2013.

16. Rosenbaum S, Shin P. Health Centers Reauthorization: an overview of achievements and challenges. 2006. Available at: http://www.kff.org/uninsured/upload/7471.pdf. Accessed December 1, 2013.

17. Robert Wood Johnson Foundation. Workforce innovations in oral health: dental professionals in non-dental settings. 2013. Available at: http://www.rwjf.org/content/dam/farm/reports/reports/2013/rwjf407852. Accessed December 1, 2013.

18. Giddon D, Swann B, Herman-Miller R. Dentists as oral physicians: the overlooked primary health care resource. J Prim Prev 2013;34(4):279–91.

19. Rosenthal R, Rosnow RL. People studying people artifacts and ethics in behavioral research. New York: Freeman; 1997.

20. American Dental Hygienists' Association. Direct Access States, 2013. Available at: http://www.adha.org/resources-docs/7513_Direct_Access_to_Care_from_DH.pdf. Accessed December 15, 2013.

21. The Pew Charitable Trusts. Growing the Dental Workforce. 2013. Available at: http://www.pewstates.org/uploadedFiles/PCS_Assets/2013/Pew_dental_workforce.pdf. Accessed December 15, 2013.

22. American Dental Hygienists' Association. Medicaid reimbursement. 2013. Available at: http://www.adha.org/reimbursement. Accessed December 15, 2013.

23. Twelve key informants, including public health dental hygienists practicing in Massachusetts. (2013, February–May) Personal interviews by phone and in person.

24. McKinnon M, Luke G, Bresch J, et al. Emerging allied dental workforce models: considerations for academic dental institutions. J Dent Educ 2007;71(11):1476–91.

25. Edelstein B. Examining whether dental therapists constitute a disruptive innovation in US dentistry. Am J Public Health 2011;101(10):1831–5.

26. Massachusetts Department of Public Health Office of Oral Health. The commonwealth's high risk senior population: results and recommendations from a 2009 statewide oral health assessment. Boston: Massachusetts Department of Public

Health; 2010. Available at: http://www.mass.gov/eohhs/docs/dph/com-health/oral-health/senior-oral-health-assessment-report.pdf.

27. Preshaw PM, Alba L, Herrera D, et al. Periodontitis and diabetes: a two-way relationship. Diabetologia 2012;55(1):21–31. http://dx.doi.org/10.1007/s00125-011-2342-y.

28. Toothwisdom. Social work and dentistry. 2013. Available at: http://www.toothwisdom.org/resources/entry/social-work-and-dentistry. Accessed November 10, 2013.

29. Noffsinger EB, Scott JC. Understanding today's group-visit models. Perm J 2000; 4(2):99–112.

30. Soderland K. Environmental scan shows dentistry entering a new normal. Chicago: ADA News; 2013. Available at: http://www.ada.org/news/9108.aspx.

31. Dolan T, Atchison K, Hyunh T. Access to dental care among older adults in the United States. J Dent Educ 2005;69(9):961–74.

32. Dounis G, Ditmyer M, McClain M, et al. Preparing the dental workforce for oral disease prevention in an aging population. J Dent Educ 2010;74(10):1086–94.

33. Coleman P, Watson N. Oral care provided by certified nursing assistants in nursing homes. J Am Geriatr Soc 2005;54:138–43.

Index

Note: Page numbers of article titles are in **boldface** type.

A

Activities of daily living, cognitive impairment and, 817, 818
Age-related changes, in body, 784
Aging, chronologic, 784
   of older adult(s), physiology of, **729–738**
   physiology of, 730
   successful, 718–719
Alzheimers disease, and dementia, 820
Anticholinergic medications, actions of, 785–787
   overcoming effects of, 792
Arthritis, definition of, 807
   drug interactions in, 807
   oral health implications of, 807
   provision of dental care in, 807–808
Aspiration pneumonia. See *Pneumonia.*
Assisted living facilities, 719

B

Bouvé College, and interdisciplinary health sciences curriculum, 833–834
Brain, healthy, definition of, and cognitive impairment, 817

C

Calcium, and phosphate, supersaturated, mucosal healing and, 793
Candidiasis, oral, 788–789
Cardiovascular changes, associated with oral health, 730–731
Cardiovascular disease, causes of, 804
   drug interactions in, 805
   oral health complications of, 805
   provision of dental care in, 806
   types of, 805
Cementum, changes in, associated with oral health, 734
Cerebrovascular disease, 806–807
Cognitive impairment, activities of daily living and, 817, 818
   communication and behavioral strategies for adults with, 822–823
   definition of healthy brain and, 817
   demographics of, 816–817
   early intervention in, 821–822
   in dementia, 819, 820
   in older adults, and oral health considerations, **815–828**
   interdisciplinarry approach to dental care in, 824

Dent Clin N Am 58 (2014) 857–862
http://dx.doi.org/10.1016/S0011-8532(14)00086-X
0011-8532/14/$ – see front matter © 2014 Elsevier Inc. All rights reserved.

dental.theclinics.com

United States Postal Service

Statement of Ownership, Management, and Circulation
(All Periodicals Publications Except Requester Publications)

1. Publication Title	2. Publication Number							3. Filing Date
Dental Clinics of North America	5	6	6	-	4	8	0	9/14/14

4. Issue Frequency	5. Number of Issues Published Annually	6. Annual Subscription Price
Jan, Apr, Jul, Oct	4	$280.00

7. Complete Mailing Address of Known Office of Publication (Not printer) (Street, city, county, state, and ZIP+4®)

Elsevier Inc.
360 Park Avenue South
New York, NY 10010-1710

Contact Person: Stephen R. Bushing
Telephone (Include area code): 215-239-3688

8. Complete Mailing Address of Headquarters or General Business Office of Publisher (Not printer)

Elsevier Inc., 360 Park Avenue South, New York, NY 10010-1710

9. Full Names and Complete Mailing Addresses of Publisher, Editor, and Managing Editor (Do not leave blank)

Publisher (Name and complete mailing address)

Linda Belfus, Elsevier Inc., 1600 John F. Kennedy Blvd., Suite 1800, Philadelphia, PA 19103-2899

Editor (Name and complete mailing address)

John Vassallo, Elsevier Inc., 1600 John F. Kennedy Blvd., Suite 1800, Philadelphia, PA 19103-2899

Managing Editor (Name and complete mailing address)

Adrianne Brigido, Elsevier Inc., 1600 John F. Kennedy Blvd., Suite 1800, Philadelphia, PA 19103-2899

10. Owner (Do not leave blank. If the publication is owned by a corporation, give the name and address of the corporation immediately followed by the names and addresses of all stockholders owning or holding 1 percent or more of the total amount of stock. If not owned by a corporation, give the names and addresses of the individual owners. If owned by a partnership or other unincorporated firm, give its name and address as well as those of each individual owner. If the publication is published by a nonprofit organization, give its name and address.)

Full Name	Complete Mailing Address
Wholly owned subsidiary of	1600 John F. Kennedy Blvd, Ste. 1800
Reed/Elsevier, US holdings	Philadelphia, PA 19103-2899

11. Known Bondholders, Mortgagees, and Other Security Holders Owning or Holding 1 Percent or More of Total Amount of Bonds, Mortgages, or Other Securities. If none, check box ☐ None

Full Name	Complete Mailing Address
N/A	

12. Tax Status (For completion by nonprofit organizations authorized to mail at nonprofit rates) (Check one)
The purpose, function, and nonprofit status of this organization and the exempt status for federal income tax purposes:
☐ Has Not Changed During Preceding 12 Months
☐ Has Changed During Preceding 12 Months (Publisher must submit explanation of change with this statement)

PS Form **3526**, August 2012 (Page 1 of 3 (Instructions Page 3)) PSN 7530-01-000-9931 **PRIVACY NOTICE:** See our Privacy policy in www.usps.com

---

13. Publication Title	14. Issue Date for Circulation Data Below
Dental Clinics of North America	July 2014

15. Extent and Nature of Circulation				Average No. Copies Each Issue During Preceding 12 Months	No. Copies of Single Issue Published Nearest to Filing Date
a. Total Number of Copies (Net press run)				958	1,028
b. Paid Circulation (By Mail and Outside the Mail)	(1)	Mailed Outside-County Paid Subscriptions Stated on PS Form 3541 (Include paid distribution above nominal rate, advertiser's proof copies, and exchange copies)		466	546
	(2)	Mailed In-County Paid Subscriptions Stated on PS Form 3541 (Include paid distribution above nominal rate, advertiser's proof copies, and exchange copies)			
	(3)	Paid Distribution Outside the Mails Including Sales Through Dealers and Carriers, Street Vendors, Counter Sales, and Other Paid Distribution Outside USPS®		197	228
	(4)	Paid Distribution by Other Classes Mailed Through the USPS (e.g. First-Class Mail®)			
c. Total Paid Distribution (Sum of 15b (1), (2), (3), and (4))			▲	633	774
d. Free or Nominal Rate Distribution (By Mail and Outside the Mail)	(1)	Free or Nominal Rate Outside-County Copies Included on PS Form 3541		57	54
	(2)	Free or Nominal Rate In-County Copies Included on PS Form 3541			
	(3)	Free or Nominal Rate Copies Mailed at Other Classes Through the USPS (e.g. First-Class Mail)			
	(4)	Free or Nominal Rate Distribution Outside the Mail (Carriers or other means)			
e. Total Free or Nominal Rate Distribution (Sum of 15d (1), (2), (3) and (4))			▲	57	54
f. Total Distribution (Sum of 15c and 15e)			▲	720	828
g. Copies not Distributed (See instructions to publishers #4 (page #3))			▲	238	200
h. Total (Sum of 15f and g)			▲	958	1,028
i. Percent Paid (15c divided by 15f times 100)				92.08%	93.48%

16. Total circulation includes electronic copies. Report circulation on PS Form 3526-X worksheet.

17. Publication of Statement of Ownership
If the publication is a general publication, publication of this statement is required. Will be printed in the October 2014 issue of this publication.

18. Signature and Title of Editor, Publisher, Business Manager, or Owner

Stephen R. Bushing – Inventory Distribution Coordinator

Date: September 14, 2014

I certify that all information furnished on this form is true and complete. I understand that anyone who furnishes false or misleading information on this form or who omits material or information requested on the form may be subject to criminal sanctions (including fines and imprisonment) and/or civil sanctions (including civil penalties).

PS Form **3526**, August 2012 (Page 2 of 3)

Moving?

Make sure your subscription moves with you!

To notify us of your new address, find your **Clinics Account Number** (located on your mailing label above your name), and contact customer service at:

Email: journalscustomerservice-usa@elsevier.com

800-654-2452 (subscribers in the U.S. & Canada)
314-447-8871 (subscribers outside of the U.S. & Canada)

Fax number: 314-447-8029

Elsevier Health Sciences Division
Subscription Customer Service
3251 Riverport Lane
Maryland Heights, MO 63043

*To ensure uninterrupted delivery of your subscription,
please notify us at least 4 weeks in advance of move.